Praise for Mana[g...]
Stress in Diffic[u...]

SIMPLE AND DIRECT

"This was the simplest, most direct, and easily understandable presentation on the subject of Shiatsu that I have encountered. The Behavioral Kinesiology was most enlightening. This applies both to your lecture/demonstration and your book.

— June Silverman
Supervisor, Therapeutic Nursing Program.
N.Y.U.–Bellevue Medical Center

IMMEDIATE RESULTS

"Your book is indeed a joy and a handbook for what ails a body (and mind!). Shiatsu does the trick for sinus headaches, and your instructions for meditation are concise: the kind of instructions that bring about immediate results. The beauty of your book is its simplicity and workability."

— B. T., Pittsburgh, Pennsylvania

OFFERS MUCH

"Jerry is dedicated to caring healing, and does his homework well and professionally. His is a quiet strength. His book offers much, and it works."

— Robert Dean Meridith, Former Dean
School of Planning and Architecture
Pratt Institute

SLEEPING BETTER

"I read your book regularly and am sleeping better. My mind is relaxed, and I can tell when my muscles are tense. Then I think of a beautiful place, and before I know it I'm fast asleep."

— P.P., Denver, Colorado

MANY WILL FIND IT USEFUL

"Your book is excellent. We have enjoyed it very much, and are sure many will find it useful also."

— Pat L. Payson, Librarian
Southwest Wisconsin Vo-Tech Institute

More Reader Comments

BEST RELAXATION IN YEARS
"My husband came home from work with a severe headache. He rarely gets one, and this was a dilly. He went straight to bed, but three hours later it was just as bad. Then I remembered an article on Shiatsu ('Push Here for Pain Relief,' an article about Jerry Teplitz which appeared in Prevention magazine, April 1980) and the pressure points for treating a headache. I followed the diagram, and the results were amazing.

"After one 'treatment,' his headache felt much better. He said he had a tingly sensation all the way down to his toes. He got up and ate dinner. Then I gave him one more treatment, and his headache was gone. He asked me to do it again because he said it felt so good–he hadn't been that relaxed in years. All from touching a few spots on his head! The next morning he woke up feeling great."

— Heather Hagaman, Flagstaff, Arizona
(Reprinted from Prevention, February 1981)

HELPS ME SLEEP
"I have begun to relax and enjoy! I like your book. I used it just the other night to learn about a tea to help me to sleep and it worked."

— D.W., San Diego, California

REALLY IMPRESSED!
"I read your book–really impressed! The meditation is a super-neat way to relax and feel good!"

— I.W., Newark, New Jersey

HIGHLY EFFECTIVE
"*Managing Your Stress In Difficult Times* is an excellent introduction to basic and practical principles of holistic health. The book is designed to get the reader to actually practice fundamental and highly effective techniques of relaxation and positive health. Highly effective, clearly written, and beautifully designed for the beginning reader."

— Robert Frager, Director
California Institute of Transpersonal Psychology

MANAGING
YOUR STRESS
IN DIFFICULT
—— TIMES ——
Succeeding in
Times of Change

Jerry V. Teplitz, J.D., Ph.D.,
Certified Speaking Professional

with Shelly Kellman

Foreword by John Diamond, M.D.
Past President, International Academy of Preventive Medicine

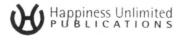
Happiness Unlimited
PUBLICATIONS

To the Spirit of Life within Us All…

HAPPINESS UNLIMITED PUBLICATIONS, Inc.
1304 Woodhurst Drive Virginia Beach, VA 23454
757.496.8008
FAX 757.496.9955
Email: Info@Teplitz.com

www.Teplitz.com

Publisher's Cataloging-in-Publication data

Teplitz, Jerry.
    Managing your stress in difficult times : succeeding in times of change /
Jerry V. Teplitz, J.D., Ph.D. ; Norma Eckroate.
    p. cm.
    Includes index.
    ISBN 978-0-939372-16-4
1. Stress management. 2. Stress (Psychology). 3. Stress (Physiology).
4. Relaxation. 5. Yoga. I. Eckroate, Norma, 1951-. II. Title.

RA785 .T46 2010
155.9042 22   2010904091

Contents

Foreword

Jerry Teplitz is doing important work. He is introducing people to natural, uncomplicated approaches to health maintenance, which are extremely valuable in the framework of holistic health. The holistic approach to medicine has a very long tradition. It is in keeping with the recorded history of medicine, of Hippocrates, Paracelsus, Maimonides. It recognizes the tremendous advances of present-day medical science, but insists on incorporating them, when appropriate, into an overall understanding and approach to the patient as a total human being, resisting the blandishments and enticements of "modern" medicine to treat the patient merely in terms of a specific disease, focusing on the "pill for every ill" approach.

Holistic medicine recognizes that a patient is at the moment of presentation to the doctor the sum total of all his life activities–his thoughts, his actions, his desires, his nutrition, his environment. Thus a total cure involves not just an alleviation of the symptoms, but also helping the individual to re-assess his life, to recognize that illness comes about because of a straying from the path of nature. It requires the recognition that the cure lies in his own hands, that he must take responsibility for the mistakes of his own existence, of which his illness is a sign.

He must recognize that some of his activities have divorced him from nature, have alienated him from his true path in life, and that it is by finding this path, by once again focusing on his true goal, that he will be cured. He must be helped to understand that the true goal of life is not what we are led to believe–material worth, evanescent pleasure, the pursuit of power–but a complete unfoldment and evolution of one's being, so that when one leaves the corporeal life there has been a progression, an evolution, an advancement of his total being, which is ultimately of benefit to those with whom he comes in contact. And this concept of personal responsibility has been thoughtfully and carefully presented in this book.

I can heartily recommend this book to you, just as I do to my own patients and students. It is an extremely well-written, concise, and comprehensive compilation of some of the most important work in many fields of natural approaches to health. You will learn more than new techniques of self help. You will, and I know this is Jerry's basic purpose, derive a new understanding of the utmost importance of an overall philosophy of positive health and positive living. The basic philosophy that he imparts is his most important contribution.

— John Diamond, M.D.
Valley Cottage, New York

Dr. Diamond is the author of Your Body Doesn't Lie; Director of the Institute of Behavioral Kinesiology; and past President of the International Academy of Preventive Medicine.

Acknowledgments

We'd like to say THANK YOU and give a great big collective hug to those people and groups that made this book possible, namely:

Swami Kriyananda and the Temple of Kriya Yoga
Belinda Lange Sweet
Jerry Spiegel and the Lakeview Educational Association
Happiness Unlimited
Gordon Seth Kramer
Maurice ("Uncle Mouse") Webster
Donna Mosher
Elizabeth Balcar
Our parents
God

AND

To those who donated time, talent, artistic skills, advice, information, or resources which made the production of this book a lot easier, namely:

Justin Pomeroy, for the chapter on herbs
Jeanne Ludwig
Sharon Glass
Karl Kristoff and Studio K
Lisa Boynton
Jon Ludwig
Patty Baker
Marcella Ruble-Rook
Al Gaspar

JoAnne Canyon-Heller
John Everest
Jonathan Phillips
Pat Yeghissian
Linda Dovey
Debbie Morkas
Carol D. Sigel
Bob Sandidge, Geoffrey Hulin, and New Orient Media

AND

To those entities which unwittingly played a part in this work:
All the businesses, associations, and universities to which Jerry has presented the "How to Relax" program The Mid-Day Live Show in New York City

Introduction

This is a very practical book. You can begin new ways of relaxing almost from the first page. The techniques in this book are easy, effective, and quick to learn. You can do them by yourself, with a friend, in a group.
I'm the kind of person who always looks for the shortest, simplest way to anything. The exercises in this book are designed to give you the greatest benefits in these difficult times with the least amount of effort or change in your routine.

Most of the material in this book has been field-tested many, many times. For more than three decades, I have been teaching seminars on meditation, yoga, Shiatsu, and nutrition at colleges and universities, at conferences, and on television and radio shows throughout the country and around the world. Thousands of people have experienced the methods presented in this book, and their response has been remarkable. Almost every single person has reported the programs to be very beneficial. This consistent positive response was one of the things that encouraged me to write this book.

Before I began teaching, I was a practicing attorney. When I began to explore these areas of relaxation, I did it with a trained lawyer's skepticism. While I was intrigued, I thought much of it was gimmicky or just not true. By trying them out for myself, I discovered the tremendous validity and worth of these techniques.

I give this book to you, the reader, not just to read, but to experience. You will almost immediately notice differences taking place in your level of relaxation. It's fine to be skeptical, but be curious, too. These are techniques that will allow you handle your stress in these times more effectively and successfully.

This book is written as a beginner-level introduction to the various subjects presented. Each chapter is complete and can be done by itself to teach you how to deal with your stress.

If one method of stress management does not appeal to you, don't close the book and walk away; just turn to another section. There is a technique that will fit just about anyone. You can compare this book to a department store—if you don't find something in house wares, you might find it in hardware.

A unique section of this book is the one on Shiatsu. Shiatsu is a Japanese finger pressure technique that is similar to acupuncture. This section includes treatments for the everyday health problems that keep you from relaxing. For example, it's hard to relax and handle your stress when your nose is stuffed up.

The nutrition section of this book is the one section from which you won't see changes instantly; however, by following the advice outlined, you will notice the changes in you and your life within a few weeks.

For me, the fulfilling part of teaching these techniques comes when I meet someone I've taught who says, "You know, I'm amazed. I tried the Shiatsu headache treatment on myself and on my friends, and it works." Or, "I've been meditating regularly and it's incredible, all the changes that have happened to me. I won't miss meditating for anything."

Just by following the simple instructions in this book, you, too, can both change and take control of your life. While external events and activities will continue to happen, it's actually your internal self that decides your reaction to these external stimuli. For example, two good friends go to see the same movie. Afterward one says, "Best movie I've ever seen," and the other says, "I didn't really like it." The external event was the same, but both had different internal reactions.

By knowing how to relax, how to energize, how to get rid of headaches or sore throats, you'll begin to consciously select how you react to a given situation. If some occurrence gets you stressed, you'll be able to do a breathing exercise. If you feel tired and dragged out, you'll be able to meditate. If you can't fall asleep, you'll be able to do the progressive relaxation exercise.

The "Body Talk" section must be tried to be believed. Everything around us has an effect on us. This section will generate a tremendous amount of excitement in you when you experience the techniques described.

Knowing that you are in control is something many people have forgotten in these times. We have been so flooded by product advertisements for this drug, that illness, or that discomfort that we've forgotten we are our own best doctors. This lack of control is best illustrated by the fact that about 80 percent of the people going to doctors are complaining of psychosomatic illnesses—illnesses caused by tension, anxiety, and feelings of an inability to cope. Dentists are even noticing more patients coming into their offices with cracked teeth due to stresses in their lives that are causing them to grind their teeth more.

This book or any section of this book will begin to give you back your rightful power and control over your mind, body, and spirit. Happy relaxing!

Chapter 1
Riding the Rapids

There's no doubt about it—times are difficult, and that's leading people to experience more and more stress. From being laid off, to losing your house, to having to work past when you planned to retire, you may be facing a difficult time yourself. Even if none of these calamities is affecting you personally, you know people who are. At a minimum, just by reading the newspapers and online reports and by watching TV news shows and listening to commentators, you're probably feeling nervous about the future.

Welcome to stress that's going on in the world today. Your experiencing all this stress is not benign either. High levels of stress can lead to high blood pressure, digestive problems, difficulty concentrating, impaired immune function, and increased risk of disease. For more than three decades, I've been pioneering ways that people can take charge of their personal energy system each and every day of their life. This book is designed to give you an experience of the stress-reduction strategies that I have studied, taught, and used myself for more than thirty-five years.

Like you, I have not been immune to experiencing the "difficult times" impacting our society. My business has required more from my staff and me, travel has become more challenging, expenses have increased…life has just demanded more! The practices you are about to learn in this book are ones that have enabled me to maintain a healthy body, a calm mind, and a much more relaxed lifestyle. I owe my vibrant well-being to these simple techniques, and I am excited to be able to share them with you. Best of all, many of these are techniques you can use immediately to reduce your level of stress, even with all the things that are going on around you.

A few years ago, I went whitewater rafting on the Gauley River in West Virginia. This is normally a Class 5 river, which means the rapids are big stuff. Because of heavy rains over the previous week, the water speed and level were three times the normal flow—just below flood levels—which meant there was "really, really big stuff" to run.

On one major rapid, I got knocked out of the boat along with three other people. Two were pulled back onto the raft. I was too far away to get back to the raft. This was a dangerous rapid because it had a place called a "hydraulic" where I could get stuck and never be able to get out. It was called Maytag because once you got into it you just went around and around.

The people on the raft started shouting franticly at me to "swim left, swim left" to avoid the hydraulic! Fortunately, my high school swim team skills kicked in, and I was able to avoid being pulled into the hydraulic by two feet. A few seconds later, I was pulled back into the raft. I was breathing hard and felt exhausted and could barely move; however, we had the next set of rapids coming up fast.

Now this was actually the part that amazed me. After a couple of deep breaths and about a minute of rest, I was back paddling again—no adrenaline rush, no-after effect shaking, no freaking out. Just doing it.

As a result of this experience, I have a new view of life as a raft trip down a whitewater river. At times things are calm and placid, and at other times we're facing a rapid. So when difficult times hit, what do you do? Do things happen in life that knock you out of your boat? Do things happen that you don't like? Do people say things that strike you the wrong way? Do you then swim as hard as you can to get back into the boat, or do you just give up and let the river take you over the rocks? When you get back in the boat of life, do you pick up your paddle again and give it half your energy, or do you give it your all?

Has your life recently been feeling like my whitewater-river experience? You're certainly not alone, of course. As I said, few of us have escaped the impact of job losses, drastic reductions in retirement accounts, or trying to balance a household budget when everything seems to cost more. At work, if you are a business owner, you may be struggling to cover expenses with less income while maintaining confidence among clients and employees. If you're an employee, you may be praying that your job stays in existence while working more hours for the same or less pay.

Stress management techniques, time management methods, healthy nutritional approaches, and exercise become even more important to include in your life to weather these storms. This book will share with you many techniques and methods that, while they may be new to you, really work.

While you may not be able to change the events that are happening to you, you still have a choice in how you personally will navigate the rapids in these difficult times. Since we are all individuals taking the ride on this raft called life, the question is: what choices are you making? You can choose to suffer and give up, or you can practice the proven techniques in this book to create smoother water inside yourself for you to ride.

Stress and Vitality

The ability to cope with stress strongly influences one's health and vitality. If not properly managed, both acute and chronic stress can negatively affect immune, enzyme, and hormone function. Marc Isaacson of the Village Green Apothecary in Bethesda, Maryland, presents some powerful statistics about the impact of stress on vitality. According to some estimates, about 80 percent of common diseases are related to prolonged stress. The Mayo Clinic reported that psychological stress is the strongest risk factor predictive of future cardiac events, including myocardial infarction and cardiac death, among individuals with existing coronary artery disease.

In addition, Isaacson says, chronic stress elevates the hormone cortisol, which can contribute to the development of metabolic syndrome, including abdominal obesity and other risk factors for diabetes and cardiovascular disease. Negative emotions and psychological stress also raise the production of proinflammatory chemicals, a risk factor for age-related diseases and conditions including cardiovascular disease, diabetes, osteoporosis, arthritis, cancer, and Alzheimer's. Because stress can dampen immune response, it can increase the risk of infection and delay wound healing.

Researchers have also found that people dramatically increase their use of the medical system during times of job insecurity, which, of course, leads to increased levels of stress. Doctor visits tend to increase by as much as 150 percent, episodes of illness increase 70 percent, and visits to hospital outpatient departments increase 160 percent. It is estimated that 75 to 90 percent of all doctor visits are due to stress related complaints; stress management could eliminate a large percentage of these visits, Isaacson suggests. And I agree.

The Impact of Stress at Work

When people lose their jobs, the remaining employees find themselves with too much to do and fewer people to help do it.

A study published a few years ago found that 44 percent of U.S. employees were overworked "often" or "very often." Those who ranked in the highly overworked category were more likely to make mistakes at work, feel angry with their employers for expecting them to do too much, resent the coworkers who didn't work as hard as they did, have higher stress levels, be depressed, have health problems, or be neglectful with respect to caring for themselves. Today, these figures are probably even higher.

A study reported in the online Journal of Occupational Environment Medicine was conducted over a ten-year period at the Karolinska Institute in Stockholm, Sweden. Researchers observed the long-term health effects that a boss might have on his or her employees. The study tracked 3,000 men with an average age of 42 and better than average access to health care. Each participant rated their boss's behavior on ten measures, including statements such as "My boss gives me the information I need" and "I have sufficient power in relation to my responsibilities."

By the end of the study, 74 men had suffered heart attacks and other serious cardiac events. It turned out that the lower a boss's leadership score, the higher the worker's risk of having a cardiac event. The chance of a heart attack also increased with the number of years of working for that bad boss.

When you are under sustained levels of stress your body secretes adrenaline, and you wind up increasing your blood pressure. This ongoing increase in blood pressure can lead to increases in heart disease because this increase in the heart's workload weakens it over time. This sustained stress can also wind up increasing the risk of stroke, heart attack, kidney failure, and congestive heart failure. Being chronically depressed can also increase risks to the heart.

A study of 33,000 men found that chronic or serious anxiety increased the likelihood of sudden cardiac death six times more than those who scored low on an anxiety symptom questionnaire. Since 200,000 men die each year, reducing a man's stress level at work is especially important.

Women are more likely to be overworked than men. While men tend to work longer hours, women experience more stress from the need to multi-task and the increased demands at both work and at home.

Women have an additional health concern caused by work-related stress if they do not have an environment in which they are free to express themselves. A study in Psychosomatic Medicine reports that middle-aged women who swallow their anger and often worry about making a good impression show biological signs that makes them more likely to have a heart attack when they are in their sixties. The researchers followed two hundred women over a ten-year period and found those who were more hostile had thicker carotid arteries, which is a sign of higher risk for coronaries and strokes. So, when you're angry, express it if it's appropriate. If not, use some of the stress management techniques in this book to calm down.

Women under stress at work can reduce their stress by finding support from other women in the workplace. Prevention magazine reported a study of women and their response to stress. There's a chemical a woman's body produces when she is under stress called oxytocin. It actually encourages the woman to take care of children and gather with other women. When she does, even more oxytocin is released, which continues to counter stress effects by producing a calming effect. This means it's important for women to have a support network of other women.

The Impact of Stress And Fatigue

In a crisis, our instincts can lead to our undoing. Research shows that when we are calm, our brains require eight to ten seconds to process each novel piece of complex information. The greater our levels of stress, the more the brain's processing time slows down. When a crisis hits, our brains will actually move into low gear just at the time when we need it to be moving faster. In response to a disaster, many people will often say to themselves: "This can't possibly be happening to me." Before deciding what to do and taking action, they will check with four or more sources, including family, news sources, and public officials.

In a disaster, ten to fifteen percent of the affected people will remain calm, acting quickly and efficiently, and fifteen percent will panic. The vast majority, however, will do very little; they are stunned and bewildered. While most people are aware that we have a flight-or-fight survival response that can get triggered in emergencies, there is also a freeze response. Freezing is what happens to a deer when caught in a car's headlights. The deer freezes, and the car hits it. When a disaster occurs, people who are stunned are actually experiencing the freeze part of the survival mechanism.

According to Mac McLean, who has been studying plane evacuations for sixteen years at the FAA's Civil Aerospace Medical Institute, there is a way to override this freeze instinct: by training and by thinking about what you would do in a disaster situation. A mental plan will give your brain a road map to follow when a disaster occurs so you won't freeze, and you will instead move to flee or fight.

For example, if you think you might lose your job, you need to begin to plan a course of action before you are in that stressful situation, so you are ready to act if you do get fired.

And don't worry about making the perfect decision. As a culture, consumers have found themselves with more and more choices on everything. Having all these choices may be making it hard for us to choose anything. A study reported in Discover magazine found that participants were able to successfully juggle four different chucks of information in any given instant. When the number was increased to five, they became confused. An AARP report supports this concern for our number of choices today. Whether it's 85 different types of crackers to choose from in a supermarket to thousands of mutual funds to select from, we are becoming overwhelmed with the choices we face when making even the simplest decisions.

Some studies have shown that as a supermarket increases the variety of products on its shelves, the number of sales actually go down. As the number of mutual funds in a 401(k) retirement plan goes up, the likelihood employees will pick any of them goes down. Even patient satisfaction goes down when the choices of medical treatments for an ailment go up. All these choices are enough to make a person depressed, and it does.

To reduce your stress, recognize that you don't have to pick the perfect strategy in these difficult times. Rather, ask yourself, "Is this choice helpful for what I need now?" Then, make a decision. Using some of the techniques in this book will make it easier for you to be adaptable and keep making decisions.

Natural Ways to Reduce Stress

While there are countless ways to reduce your level of stress, this book explores specific techniques that have helped hundreds of thousands of people to reduce their stress and eliminate stress-related pain in their bodies. These are very simple things you can begin to do that will bring you stress relief. Just pay attention to your body. For example, have you been sitting at you desk for so long that you're not able to think clearly? Taking a twenty-minute walk will bring you immediate relief.

I was pleased when I read that taking that walk in a nature environment had an even more positive impact. Studies have shown that vegetation and green spaces in a community can strengthen social ties, reduce levels of aggression and violence, cause crime rates to drop, and even help reduce people's stress. One study even found that kids interacting with nature experienced significant reductions in their attention deficit disorder symptoms. Also, it reported, a view of nature from the bedroom window gave girls a greater ability to concentrate, and it even increased their self-discipline.

Have you been avoiding someone or something important that is creating stress because you just don't want to think about it? Well, think about it! A study at Case Western Reserve University found that ignoring someone requires a lot of mental energy. The researchers put a student in a room with a research team member for four minutes. Half the students were told to ignore their partner and half were told to talk to them. Later the researchers gave each student twenty word puzzles to do. Those who talked to their partner were more persistent in their efforts to solve the puzzles than those who ignored their partners. When you're having a problem with a friend or family member, it may be better for your health while reducing your stress level to talk the situation out than attempt to ignore it.

And here's another idea: Consider increasing your social interaction through volunteering—even just one hour a week. People who volunteered for that amount of time experienced a 30 percent lower mortality rate.

Your mind is willing to support you in slowing down and reducing the stress in your life. Ask it for support and to give you opportunities in your environment to relax.

I should know. The amount of marketing, management time, and travel my work requires makes me an ideal candidate for high levels of stress. So, for more than thirty-five years I've made myself a living stress management experiment by doing the things I teach to obtain optimum wellness. I exercise, practice yoga, meditate, take vitamins and minerals, eat a vegetarian diet, maintain a positive attitude, attend church regularly, and do work that I enjoy.

As proof, I recently had my yearly visit to my doctor. My blood pressure was 106 over 68 and my pulse was 60 beats per minute. My PSA was 1.3. My cholesterol was 153.

And—best of all—I just turned 62! This stuff works. All you need is to just do it!

I invite you to join me in this experience in managing your stress, no matter how tough life seems to be. Sit back, relax, and read about how these very specific, very effective techniques can ease your stress, regardless of how rough the rapids get on this whitewater river we call life. Enjoy the ride!

Chapter 2
Breathing

In Hatha Yoga, there is a principle called pranayama, meaning breath. In yoga, breath is viewed as the primary life force. This makes sense when one realizes that we can do without food and water for long periods of time, but we can only do for a very short period (three to six minutes) without breathing.

Pranayama is also a way to relax totally and completely. Have you ever stopped to notice your breathing when you're scared or startled? It would be short and shallow. Slowing your breath activates the parasympathetic nervous system, which helps lower heart rate, perspiration and other physical signs of stress. Any time you feel fear or tension, you can change that feeling simply by changing your breath rate to very long deep breaths.

Studies show that the most significant factor in health and longevity is how well you breathe. Hypertension can be controlled by the way we breathe. Properly oxygenating the body has a direct impact on the nervous system, corrects energetic balances, and impacts the body's subtle energy systems. Breathing exercises both relieve stress and work as a natural tranquilizer for the nervous system. Best of all, you can do these exercises anytime and anywhere!

I have used breathing exercises when scheduled to appear in court when I actively practiced as an attorney. To relieve tension before approaching the judge, I would do a breathing exercise. In a minute or two, I'd be calm and prepared to face the courtroom battle.

Deep Breathing

1. Sit upright, spine straight but not straining.
2. Close your eyes. (If you're in a situation where this would be inappropriate, you can keep them open.)
3. Exhale forcefully all the air in your lungs.
4. Inhale through the nose to a slow count of eight, filling first your stomach. 1...2...3...4...let it expand...then your chest... 5...6...7...and finally your shoulder blade region...8.
5. Exhale through the nose to a slow count of eight, emptying first your shoulder blades 1...2... then the chest...3...4 ...5...and finally the stomach...6...7...8. Imagine you are a balloon deflating slowly through a pinhole.
6. Repeat this process at least two more times.
7. Sit quietly with eyes closed for a minute or two. Feel how your body is relaxing.

The deep breathing exercise is easy to do any time and any place—on a bus, in a train, in a cafeteria, before a business meeting, or taking an exam. For homemakers, it is a refreshing addition to morning breaks. Some athletes habitually do deep breathing and alternate breathing between breaks in the action.

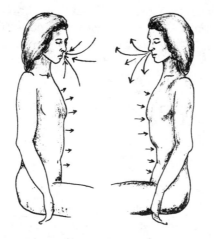

Step 4   **Step 5**

Alternate Breathing

1. Close your eyes. Sit upright, spine straight but not straining.
2. Press your left nostril closed with your right ring finger and little finger.
3. Inhale slowly (so you can barely feel your breath coming in) through your right nostril.
4. Release your left nostril. Use your thumb to close off your right nostril.
5. Now exhale slowly through your left nostril.
6. Keep your fingers in position. Inhale very slowly through your left nostril.
7. Close off your left nostril with your ring finger and little finger; release your thumb from your right nostril.
8. Now exhale slowly through your right nostril.
9. Continue doing this for at least three to five rounds.
10. Sit quietly with your eyes closed and your hands in your lap for a few minutes.

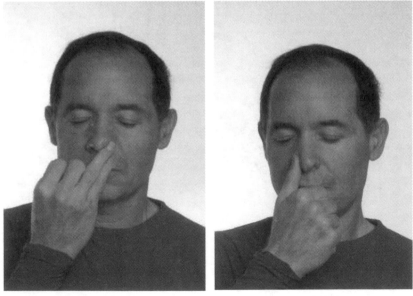

Steps 1,2,3   **Steps 4,5,6**

Cooling Breath

The cooling breath is excellent to use in hot weather. As you take the first breath, you will feel a cool sensation in your mouth. After repeating it six to fifteen times, you will feel the coolness spreading through your entire body. This exercise will also help reduce fevers.

1. Stick your tongue out with the edges curled up. Don't strain, but stick it out all the way.
2. Inhale air through the mouth, along the center of the tongue, and make a sucking sound. "Sssstthh…"
3. When you have a full abdomen of air, swallow.
4. Exhale gently through your nostrils.
5. Repeat six to fifteen It might look funny but it works. times. Relax and enjoy the cooling sensations.

(Note: Some people cannot curl their tongues properly to do this exercise.)

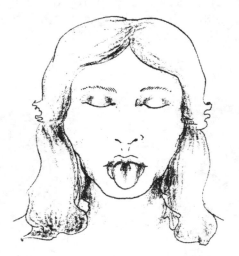

Chapter 3
Shiatsu

Shiatsu is a pressure point massage technique that's been around for several thousand years. It was formalized in the 1930s by Tokujiro Namikoshi, who founded the Nippon Shiatsu School in Japan.

Shiatsu probably came about when people in ancient times in Japan noticed that we naturally tend to rub a part of the body that is hurting. They also noted the effectiveness of the Chinese technique of acupuncture, which inserts needles into specific body points to promote healing. These principles were combined into a form now called Shiatsu, literally meaning "finger pressure."

It can be used to treat many different kinds of pain and illnesses, including: headaches, migraine headaches, sore throats and strep throats, sinus colds, eyestrain, hangovers, backaches, stiff necks, sore shoulders, and menstrual pain. These are the treatments in this chapter. Some of the treatments are also great for general relaxation and massage.

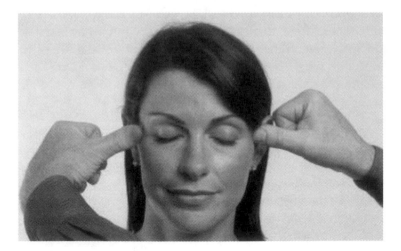

There are several theories as to why Shiatsu works:

1. It increases the flow of blood to the area pressed. The blood carries off wastes from all the cells and brings fresh oxygen, nutrients, hormones, antibodies, and white blood cells to the area.
2. Like acupuncture, Shiatsu pressure stimulates the nerve endings and meridians (energy pathways) of the body so that the body will heal itself.
3. In physics there's a principle that every action has an equal and opposite reaction. When you press on a point you contract the area, then when you release it, the muscles and blood vessels in that area stretch, expand, and relax.
4. When there's pain or tension in muscles, Shiatsu relaxes and loosens them—not only at the point pressed, but in the surrounding area. This is akin to a pebble making ripples on a lake. The pebble dropped in one spot makes ripples over a large surface of the water. Unlike the lake, however, our muscles need to be pressed on several points, with repetition, before relaxation comes about.
5. Endorphins, natural pain suppressants secreted in the brain, may be stimulated by Shiatsu pressure.

If Shiatsu is done properly, pain will disappear or be greatly reduced. This is true even for injuries, such as sprains, and certain infections like strep throat. I'm not suggesting Shiatsu as a replacement for seeing a doctor. The treatments in this section are aimed at conditions for which people do not usually seek medical help right away. Rather, the person will reach for some aspirin, a cold tablet, or a pain reliever. Shiatsu is both safer and more effective than any of these drugs. You ingest no chemicals, and the benefits are immediate. If you try Shiatsu several times during a day and feel no relief, then you know you should see a doctor.

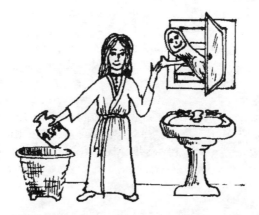

The Evidence For Shiatsu

There is plenty of evidence supporting the effectiveness of this ancient Japanese finger pressure technique. Research published in Acupuncture Electrotherapy Research more than a decade ago compared the impact of acupuncture, Shiatsu, and lifestyle adjustments in 69 patients with severe angina pectoris (chest pain). Of these, 49 were candidates for coronary artery bypass grafting surgery (CABG). The researchers compared the results with a large group of patients that did go through CABG. The incidence of death among the CABG patients was 21 percent, while the patients undergoing acupuncture and Shiatsu had a death rate of 7 percent. Sixty-one percent of the acupuncture and Shiatsu patients were able to cancel surgery due to clinical improvement. The annual number of in-hospital days was reduced by 90 percent. Interestingly, even though the men in the study reported significantly lower positive expectations toward the outcome of the study, there was no difference in the effects on men or women at the conclusion of the study.

Another study published in the Journal of Holistic Nursing validated the benefit of Shiatsu on lower back pain. In the study, 66 people who complained of lower back pain received four Shiatsu treatments. After each treatment, the subjects were called and asked to quantify the level of pain. The researchers found that both pain and anxiety decreased significantly over time.

A study published in the International Journal of Palliative Nursing reported the results of the use of Shiatsu therapy on clients attending hospice day services. Over a five-week period, even clients with advanced progressive diseases received one Shiatsu session per week. Four interviews were conducted before, during, and after the five weeks of treatment. A fifth interview was conducted four weeks after the treatments ended. The participants reported significant improvements in energy levels, relaxation, confidence, symptom control, clarity of thought, and mobility. Some benefits lasted a few hours, and others lasted past the five weeks of treatments.

A study conducted by the Touch Research Institute found that out of twelve people who were massaged thirty minutes twice per week for five weeks, 60 percent enjoyed an entire month migraine-free as opposed to only 40 percent of the controls. My experience over thirty years is that with Shiatsu you can get rid of a migraine in five minutes. While this study shows that regular massage can reduce the frequency of a migraine, Shiatsu can quickly solve the problem when it flares up. I've also had very positive feedback from migraine sufferers that have used my Shiatsu treatment. They have told me that their persistent migraines became infrequent attacks after repeating the Shiatsu treatment a number of times.

An example of Shiatsu's effectiveness: I once taught 300 skeptical convention-goers at one time how to do Shiatsu on each other for headaches (it works for hangovers, too). They had never heard of it before. At the beginning, I asked, "How many people in here have a headache?" About thirty raised their hands. After I taught the treatment and they'd done it on each other, I asked, "How many of you still have a headache?" Not one hand went up.

Determining The Correct Shiatsu Pressure

The correct Shiatsu pressure is described as a cross between pleasure and pain. You should exert a good, hard, steady pressure on each point. Use your thumbs as much as possible. The biggest mistake most people make is not pressing hard enough.

When you are treating another person, use that person's "ouch reflex" as a pressure guide. Tell the person to say "ouch" immediately if he or she feels pain. Then let go immediately and press on the next point. Interestingly, a person may feel pain at one point and one inch away feel no pain at all, even though the pressure is the same.

So, work with the same intensity on each point, and let the person you're working on judge when the pressure is too hard. When a person does say "ouch," make a mental note of the location of that point. Then, on the second time through the treatment, when you come to the location of the "ouch" point, begin by pressing it very gently. Slowly build the pressure up. You'll be pressing for longer than usual since it's a building pressure rather than a steady one. Surprisingly, you may be able to apply more pressure than the first time around, without causing pain.

Another way to experience the kind of pressure you should be using is to place your thumb on a bathroom scale and lean on it until it registers fifteen to twenty pounds.

You can do Shiatsu on others or on yourself. Like breathing and meditation, it's a handy stress reduction tool to carry with you, requiring no special equipment and very little time. For example, the headache cure can be effectively performed in less than two minutes.

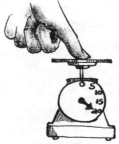

When working on yourself, it may be hard to get a good strong pressure with your thumb on some points, for instance, at the top of your head. When that occurs, put your middle finger on top of your index fingernail and press, as shown in diagram A. Or try pressing with the flat of your index finger, supported by your thumb, as in diagram B. Don't use your knuckle, just the pad of your finger.

These alternate ways of pressing are also useful when you're doing a lot

A 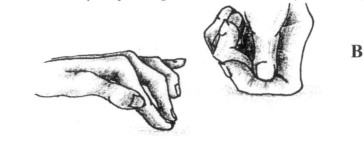 **B**

of Shiatsu on other people as a way to give your thumbs a rest.

When doing a treatment, go through all the points at least twice, even three times if the person still feels pain or discomfort. On yourself, do the treatment three or four times through since you're exerting a little less pressure than when you do it on someone else. After three or four times through the points, it's best to wait an hour or so before doing another to let the body respond. If needed, Shiatsu can be done with complete safety, over and over again.

Follow the diagrams to learn the Shiatsu points, but don't worry about pressing each point's location exactly. The body has a sympathetic and parasympathetic area surrounding each nerve ending. By pressing in the vicinity of the nerve ending, you are stimulating that nerve ending to transmit the healing message to the proper body part. That is why Shiatsu points don't have to be "hit"

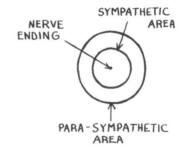

as accurately as acupuncture points, in which the needle must be inserted into an exact spot. Unless otherwise noted, Shiatsu instructions in this book are written for the person who is "treating" or working on another person. Occasionally there will be parenthetical statements about what to do differently when you are working on yourself.

Instructions on your position and which hand to use when treating someone are written for right-handed people. Left-handed persons can simply reverse the side they stand on and the hand they use, if that's more comfortable. When only one hand is involved, you'll want to press with your stronger hand.

Headaches and Hangovers

Did you know that headache and migraine medications can actually cause a headache? That's right, the very drugs people take to get rid of a headache or migraine can bring them back. Doctors call it the rebound effect. When you take pain relievers on a regular basis for more than two or three days each week, the drugs can make the pain receptors more sensitive than usual. This means when the pain medicine wears off, these hypersensitive receptors turn on to produce a new headache or migraine. You're then going down the slippery slope of more pain medicines followed by more headaches and migraines. To stop this vicious cycle you have to stop the medicine, which means you may experience a severe and painful detoxification that will last for about three days.

Dr. Fred Sheftell, the director and founder of The New England Center for Headache, believes the situation to be so serious that he says even medicine like aspirin and acetaminophen, which can trigger this rebound effect, should have labels warning of the rebound effect.

One of the benefits of Shiatsu is that it can reduce and even eliminate the need for prescription drugs and over-the-counter pain relievers. Shiatsu techniques will alleviate a headache or even a hangover in 90 seconds, and it will stop a migraine in five minutes!

The Headache and Hangover Treatment

A remarkable 90-second cure, also great for overall relaxation, this treatment can help chronic headache sufferers by reducing the frequency and severity of their headaches.

The treatment also works on hangovers because a hangover is caused by constriction of the blood vessels. When alcohol enters the body, the blood vessels open wider. Then when the alcohol is gone, the vessels react by tightening up, constricting circulation so much that it's painful. The more you've had to drink, the more violently your blood vessels will react.

Shiatsu opens up the blood vessels, restoring circulation and relieving pain quickly. It's much safer and more effective than the traditional morning-after drink, which doesn't get the body back to normal.

Press each point three seconds.

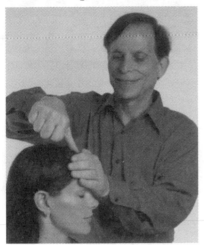

Steps 1,2

1.   The person should be seated upright, glasses off, eyes closed, in a comfortable position.

2.   Stand on the left side of the person. Support the forehead with your left hand. (No support needed when working on yourself.) With the fleshy part of your right thumb—the ball of the thumb—press at the hairline, in the center of the forehead. Move backward one inch and press again.

3.   Continue pressing points about an inch apart in a straight line, from the hairline to the hollow at the base of the skull. The hollow is the medulla oblongata. Press it also. (When working on yourself, if these points are hard to reach, remember to use the alternate methods shown on page.)

4.   Move slightly to the front of the person. Position your thumbs at the very top of the head, the highest point. Press with your thumbs, going down inch by inch on both sides, simultaneously, to the front middle of the ears.

5.   Stand to the person's left side again. Now you'll be using your right thumb and middle finger, working at the back of the head. (On yourself, use both thumbs.)

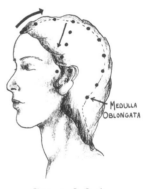

Steps 2,3,4

Find the middle of each ear. From there, go straight in toward the medulla, 1 1/2 to 2 inches on each side. There you'll find a pair of lumps, little nodes. Press them simultaneously with thumb and middle finger. Move half the distance in toward the medulla on each side. Press. Then place your thumb on the medulla and press.

6.   Come down the neck 1/2 inch from the medulla. Place thumb and middle finger on both sides of the spinal column, about an inch apart. (On yourself, use both thumbs.) Don't press on the spinal

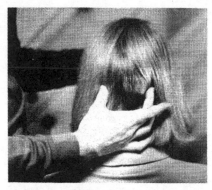

Step 5

column; press right next to it on both sides.

7. Press three or four pairs of points, depending on how long the neck is. Just go straight down; points are an inch apart. Stop at the shoulders.

8. Repeat the entire process to make one treatment. If the pain has not disappeared, go through the points a third time.

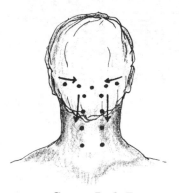

Steps 5, 6, 7

Migraine Headaches

Anyone who has had a migraine headache or has been around a migraine victim knows the pain and complete helplessness of the sufferer. Shiatsu offers almost instant relief from this problem.

I've done the Shiatsu migraine treatment with amazing success on a number of people who suffered from chronic migraines. One person I was called to work on had collapsed from the pain. She needed to be carried into the bedroom. I worked on her for about ten minutes. Twenty minutes later, she was downstairs cooking dinner.

Another time, I was at a convention and treated a delegate right in the middle of the luncheon banquet. The head of his delegation had approached me, saying that this man had been walking around all day with a headache, and that he was shouting and hitting others. When the man came to my table, I asked him if he had a migraine. He said yes, so I did the migraine treatment. In a few minutes his migraine was gone.

If you have experienced a migraine headache, you know the pain and complete helplessness you feel. Let's begin by looking more closely at migraines and the myths and truths surrounding them:

Myth: Migraines are just bad headaches.

Truth: Migraines are far worse than a bad headache. They are characterized by throbbing head pain, nausea, and sensitivity to light and sound. Attacks can last from four to 72 hours. Also, if both your parents have experienced migraines, there is a 75 percent chance that you will have them, too. If it's one parent, then the odds are 50 percent. Even if a distant relative has them, the odds are 20 percent you'll get them.

Myth: I'll know a migraine if I get one, and over-the-counter drugs will fix it.

Truth: The research shows that half of all people who get migraines have not been properly diagnosed by a doctor, whether it's because they haven't gone to a doctor or the doctor missed the diagnosis. If doctors can't make an accurate diagnose, then the likelihood of your diagnosing it is very low. If the store-bought pain or allergy medication you are taking isn't working to decrease headache pain, talk to your doctor.

Myth: Migraines are caused by stress and other psychological problems.

Truth: While it's not the cause of a migraine, stress may trigger a migraine. Doctors now realize that migraines are a neurological disorder and not a psychological one. Scientists now believe that the intense pain of a migraine attack is a result of inflammation caused by an interaction between the main sensory nerve of the brain and the brain's blood vessels.

Myth: Before a migraine starts, you will see an aura.

Truth: Not everyone experiences visual symptoms before a migraine. Only a third of migraine sufferers see an aura beforehand. If you do experience visual symptoms or auras, they may show up fifteen minutes to an hour before the migraine hits.

Myth: Avoiding certain foods, like chocolate, can cure a migraine.

Truth: You may be able to reduce the frequency of migraines by avoiding anything that triggers them, but eliminating these foods won't stop you from having any migraines.

The Migraine Headache Treatment

Press each point three seconds. The person should sit upright, with glasses off and eyes closed.

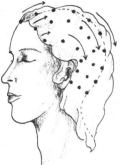

1. Stand on the left side of the person. Support the forehead with your left hand. (No support needed when working on yourself.) With the fleshy part of your right thumb, press at the hairline, in the center of the forehead.

2. Move back one inch and press again. Continue pressing points about an inch apart in a straight line, from the hairline to the hollow at the base

Steps 1,2,3,4

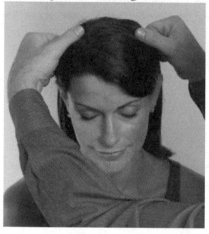

of the skull. The hollow is called the medulla oblongata. Press it, also. (When working on yourself, if these points are hard to reach, remember to use the alternate methods for applying pressure shown on page.)

3. Find the center of the hairline again and drop down one inch on each side, toward the temples. With both thumbs, press backward along the sides of the head, keeping parallel to the center line of the head. Stop when you are next to the medulla.

Step 4

4. Return to the center of the hairline and drop down two inches on each side toward the temple. Again follow an imaginary line backward along both sides of the head, skipping an inch between points, until you are in line with the medulla. (If the person has a large head, drop down a third inch from the center line and follow the same sequence.)

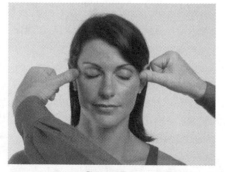

Step 5

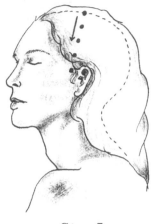

Step 5

5. Move slightly toward the front of the person. Position your thumbs at the very top of the head, the highest point. Press with your thumbs, going down inch by inch on both sides simultaneously, to the front middle of the ears.

6. Stand to the person's left again. Now you'll be using your right thumb and middle finger, working at the back of the head. (On yourself, use both thumbs.) Find the middle of each ear. From there, go straight in toward the medulla, 1 1/2 to 2 inches on each side. There you'll find a pair of lumps, little nodes. Press them simultaneously with thumb and middle finger.

7. Move half the distance in toward the medulla on each side. Press. Then place your thumb on the medulla and press.

8. Come down the neck 1/2 inch from the medulla. Place thumb and middle finger on both sides of the spinal column, about an inch apart. (On yourself, use both thumbs.) Don't press on the spinal column; press right next to it on both sides, simultaneously.

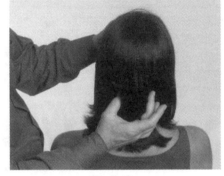

Step 7

9. Press three to five pairs of points, depending on how long the neck is. Just go straight down; points are an inch apart. Stop at the shoulders.

10. Now stand on the person's right. Support the back of the head with your left hand. (No support needed on yourself.) With your right thumb and middle finger, pinch in at the bridge of the nose. Press fingers toward each other.

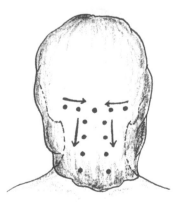

Steps 6,7,8,9

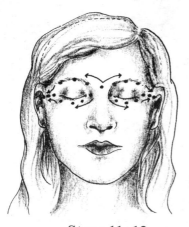

Steps 11, 12

11. Follow the lower eye bone, pressing directly on the bone, skipping an inch between points. Do both eyes at the same time, using your thumb and middle finger, until you get to the outer corners of the eyes. Using both thumbs, press just behind the outer corners of the eyes, pressing your thumbs inward, toward each other. Continue moving straight back by inches—only one or two points—until you are next to the ears.

12. At the point between the eyebrows, press in, toward the back of the head, with your right thumb. With the thumb and middle finger, follow the eyebrows, skipping an inch at a time, to the outer corners of the eyes. Switch to both thumbs and press points from the outer corners of the eyes back to the ears—only one or two points—until you reach the ears.

Do this entire process at least twice. Then ask the person how she or he feels. If the pain is greatly relieved, but not gone,

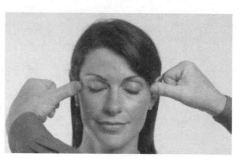

Step 11

repeat the process a third time. If the person says that the pain is now localized, just work directly on and around the pain area. Press the same points on the opposite side of the head, even if there is no pain there. You continue to work with a migraine victim until the pain is gone or you've done the treatment four or five times.

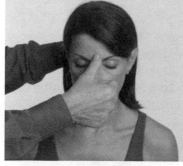

Step 12

Sinus Colds

This treatment works when the front of the face feels clogged up, with pressure around the eyes, cheeks, etc. Twice through the points is a complete treatment. After this, ask the person how he/ she feels. Most people will be able to breathe again by then. If there's still pressure or congestion, do the points a third time. The person will feel the cold breaking up and draining. If discomfort persists, wait an hour or two and do the treatment again. Keep repeating the process every hour or two until the sinus cold is gone.

Press each point three seconds. Have the person close his/her eyes.

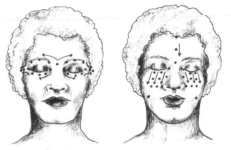

Steps 1,2,3   **Steps 4-5-6-7-8**

1. Stand on the person's right. Support the back of the head with your left hand. (No support needed on yourself.) With your right thumb and middle finger, pinch in at the bridge of the nose, pressing the fingers toward each other.
2. Follow the lower eye bone, pressing directly on the bone, skipping an inch between points. Do both eyes at the same time, using your thumb and middle finger, until you get to the outer corners of the eyes.
3. Using both thumbs, press just behind the outer corners of the eyes, pressing your thumbs inward, toward each other. Continue moving straight back an inch at a time, pressing your thumbs toward each other until you are next to the ears.
4. At the point between the eyebrows, press in with your thumb toward the back of the head. With thumb and middle finger, press the same points on the eyebrows, skipping an inch at a time, to the outer corners of the eyes. Switch to both thumbs and press points from the outer corners of the eyes back to the ears, as in step 2.
5. At the center of the hairline, press with your thumb. Press a point halfway down from hairline to the eyebrow bone. Then press directly on the eyebrow bone, just above the nose. (For steps 6 and 7, continue using the thumb and middle finger of the right hand simultaneously on both sides of the face.)

6. Pinch in at the bridge of the nose, pressing the thumb and middle finger inward toward each other. Then go down half the distance to the nostril openings and press toward the back of the head. The next point is immediately beside the nostril openings; press toward the back of the head.

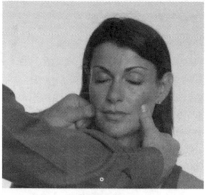

Step 9

7. Return to the lower eye bones, just below the eye sockets, only 1/2 inch outward from the bridge of the nose. Press toward the back of the head. Then drop straight down, halfway to the nostril openings and press; then go down till you're even with the nostril openings and press.

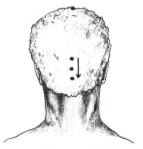

Steps 10, 11

8. Back to the eye bones. This time, start about an inch outward from the bridge of the nose. Press the same three-point sequence as in step 6, but an inch away from the nose.

9. Find the cheekbones and drop down into the hollows below. Press both sides with your thumbs right in the hollows, pressing them inward, toward each other.

10. Find the crown (top) of the head and press downward.

11. Move to the person's other side. Support the forehead with your left hand. (Not necessary when treating yourself.) Find the medulla oblongata. This is the hollow at the base of the skull, just above the neck. Move directly up the head two inches. Press. Go back down one inch and press. Go down one more inch back to the medulla, and press it.

Twice through all the steps is one treatment. You may need to go through the steps again to bring additional relief.

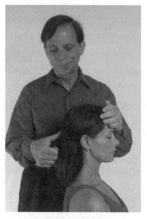

Step 11

Eye Strain

Too much reading, staring at a computer screen, playing with your iPhone, or watching television can make your eyes hurt. Here is a treatment that you can do in about one minute to relieve tension, strain, or fatigue in the eyes.

Press each point three seconds. The eyes should be closed.

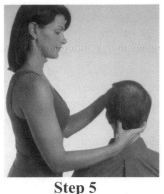

Step 5

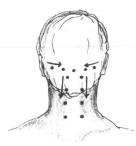

Steps 5,6

1-4. Follow instructions 1 through 4 and accompanying illustrations for the Sinus Cold Treatment, page 25.

5. Move to the person's left. Now you'll be working at the back of the person's head, using your right thumb and middle finger. (On yourself, use both thumbs.) Find the middle of each ear. From there, go straight in 1 1/2 to 2 inches on each side, toward the medulla. (This is the hollow at the base of the skull.) You'll find a pair of lumps, little nodes. Press them simultaneously with thumb and middle finger. If you can't find the lumps, so long as you are close to them, the treatment will still work.

Move inward on each side, half the distance to the medulla. Press. Then place your thumb on the medulla and press.

6. Come down the neck one-half inch from the medulla. Place your thumb and middle finger on both sides of the spinal column, about an inch apart. (On yourself, use both thumbs.) Don't press on the spinal column; press right next to it on both sides.

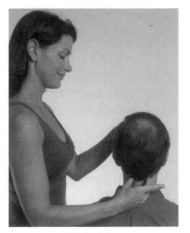

Step 6

Press three to five pairs of points, depending on how long the neck is. Just go straight down; points are an inch apart. Stop at the shoulders.

7. Repeat the entire process at least once.

Lower Back Treatment

Yes, you can get rid of your own backaches! This treatment will get rid of or greatly relieve lower back pain, strain, and fatigue. You can do it sitting up, laying down, or even standing.

These instructions are written for you to use on yourself. Before doing this on someone else, read step 1 of "Better Than a Massage," page.

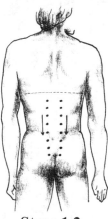

Steps 1,2

Press from three to seven seconds at each point.

1. Begin at the fifth lumbar vertebra. To find it, divide the back in half, horizontally, and drop down two inches from the center line. Don't press directly on the spine. Press on both sides of the spine simultaneously, using your thumbs.

2. Move down alongside the spine, pressing points an inch apart, until you've pressed beside the tailbone.

3. Find the place where the spine and the hipbone meet. Pressing both sides simultaneously with your thumbs, follow the hipbone outward for four pairs of equally spaced points.

4. Return to the place where the spine and the hipbone meet. The next four points form an inverted V to the middle of the buttocks.

5. Find the upper, outer portion of the buttocks and press both sides simultaneously.

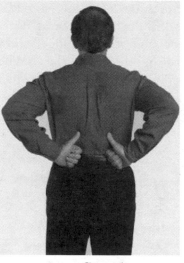

Step 1

6. Move to the lower, outer portion of the buttocks and press both sides simultaneously.

7. Repeat all steps at least once more. If there is still pain or stiffness, do it again.

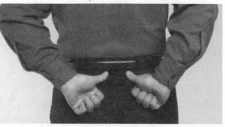

Step 3

28

To receive an extensive report on understanding, preventing and treating lower back pain you can go to this link to my website at http://linkbee. com/ReportBack.

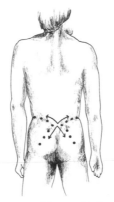

Steps 3,4

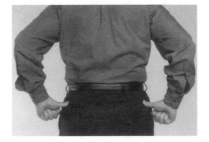

Step 5

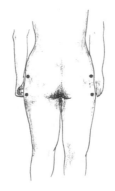

Steps 5,6

Menstrual Pain

Yes, there is something you can do about menstrual pain—your own or someone else's. This treatment brings relief without drugs. You can do the treatment on yourself, or have someone else do it for you. The cramps will disappear. If they return a few hours later, just repeat the treatment.

Press each point three to five seconds.

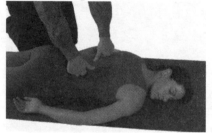

Steps 1,2

1.   Have the person lie face down. Position yourself on her left. Press all points with the thumbs, keeping arms straight and elbows locked.
2.   Find the outer ends of the lowest rib. Move straight in toward the spinal column. From this point on the spine, move your fingers up about 2 inches toward the head. This is approximately the first lumbar vertebra. Press right next to the spine (not on it) simultaneously on both sides. Next, move your fingers back down the spine until they are in line with the lowest rib. Press.

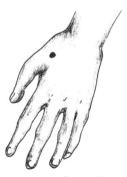

Step 6

3.   Find where the hipbone and spine meet. Move down 1 inch and press next to the spine.
4.   Find the tailbone (the very bottom of the spine.) Move up one inch and press along both sides of the spine. Move down 1/4 of an inch and press.

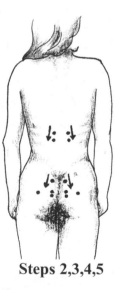

Steps 2,3,4,5

5.   From that point, move your fingers outward about 2 inches. This point should feel fleshier. If it still feels bony, move outward a little more. Press on both sides.
6.   On the back of the left hand, press the point between the thumb and index finger.

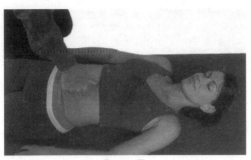

Step 7

7. Have the person lie on her back. Find the navel and move up about 3 or 4 inches to a point midway between the navel and the diaphragm. Press.

8. From the navel, drop down 1 inch and press.

9. From the navel, drop down 3 inches and press.

10. From the navel, drop down 2 inches and then move outward 2 inches on each side. Press both sides simultaneously.

11. From the navel, drop down 4 inches and then move outward 1 inch. Press both sides. Next, move back inward 1 inch and press.

12. On both legs, find the kneecap. Move upward 2 inches, then over 1 inch toward the insides of the thighs. Press.

13. Find the back middle of the calf muscle. Move 1 inch inward on the inner side of the muscles, and press both legs.

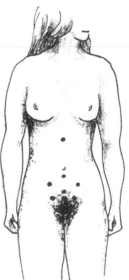

Steps 7,8,9,10,11

14. Find the inner anklebone on both legs and move up 3 inches on the inside of each leg. Press.

15. Find the inner anklebone, and press the point behind it toward the rear of the body on each leg. Press.

Repeat the entire treatment one to two times.

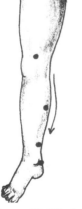

Steps 12,13-14-15

The Body's Natural Purification Plant

We can understand how Shiatsu works on sore throats, colds, and other infections by understanding the lymphatic system—our natural internal filtering and purifying plant.

The lymphatic system is a network of vessels, larger intersection points (the lymph nodes), and the fluid (lymph) that flows through the vessels. Although it is located almost parallel to the circulatory system, it functions quite differently. The system's three main jobs are:

1. Return protein that leaks out of body cells (a normal occurrence) to the blood vessels, which return it to the cells.
2. Absorb and breaks down harmful bacteria, toxins, foreign matter, and certain waste particles into harmless substances. Specialized cells found mainly in the lymph nodes perform this function. (Imagine them as waste treatment centers.)
3. Manufacture antibodies to protect the body against infection, and fight off infection once it's there. Specialized cells along the walls of the lymphatic vessels do this; the lymph carries the antibodies to the bloodstream.

How fast all of these functions are performed depends on how fast the lymph goes through the vessels. The lymph circulates around the body, collecting the wastes and foreign matter from tissues, carrying them through the filtering cells, and delivering "clean" products and antibodies into the bloodstream via the capillaries.

Unlike the circulatory system with its heart, however, the lymphatic system has no pumping mechanism. What keeps it going? Two things: one is the fluid pressure between all the body cells, and the other is simple muscle movement. It is the latter that interests us in Shiatsu.

Every time a muscle stretches or contracts anywhere in the body, it squeezes the lymphatic vessels, causing the lymph to flow faster throughout the body. The more muscle activity, the faster the lymph flows.

The Shiatsu treatments for sore throats and colds put direct pressure on the lymphatic vessels, lymph nodes, and muscles. This hard Shiatsu pressure is speeding up the lymphatic flow. This means:

1. More protein is returned to all the body cells.
2. More invading bacteria, toxins, and waste particles are cleaned out and broken down.
3. Antibodies get into the bloodstream faster.

You may have noticed that your sore throats are sometimes accompanied by "swollen glands"—tender, painful lumps on your neck beneath the hinges of your jaw. These are actually swollen lymph nodes, swollen because they've got a lot more work to do when there's an infection nearby. Shiatsu pressure on the area helps this system perform better, helping the body to heal itself naturally.

Sore Throat, Streptococcic Throat, Laryngitis, "Smoker's Throat"

A complete treatment (twice through the entire sequence) will either cure a sore throat or greatly relieve the pain. On strep throat, the treatment must be done several times a day, up to once an hour if needed. For smoker's throat, this treatment will reduce the closed-up feeling and help drain out phlegm.

Laryngitis may require up to one treatment an hour before improvement is felt. However, I once did this treatment on a film company executive with an acute case of laryngitis. By the end of the three-minute process, she was shocked to find herself speaking normally and painlessly.

The treatment is also beneficial before giving a speech or singing.

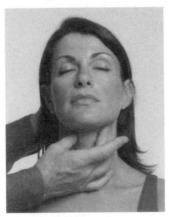

Step 1

You don't necessarily press more lightly on a throat than on a head; let the person's "ouch" be your guide. (For further explanation, see page 16.)

Press each point three seconds.
1. Stand on the right side of the person you're working on. Support the back of the head with your left hand. (Not necessary on yourself.) The center of the throat, from chin to chest, is protected by a tube of cartilage, which is bony material. Using your right hand, gently feel the throat to find where the cartilage ends. To locate the first point, move upward to where the throat and jaw connect, and press with thumb and middle finger along both sides of the cartilage. Press straight back, toward the back of the neck.

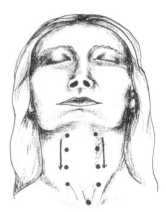

Steps 1,2

When doing the treatment on a person more than 45 years old, press on one side of the throat at a time. Drop down an inch, following the cartilage and pressing right next to it–not directly on it. The third and fourth points are called "coughing points." Widen the distance between your thumb and middle finger slightly and press. If the person coughs, move your fingers apart a bit more. The fifth point is the hollow area at the bottom of the throat by the breastbone. Use your thumb to press straight down on the bone toward the floor.

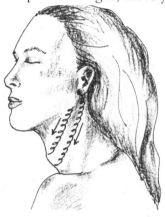

Step 3

2. Repeat step one two more times.

3. Stand in front of the person. On each hand, put your middle and index fingers together. You're going to do a circular massage at an angle down both sides of the throat. Start just behind the jaw and do small circles down to the sides of the Adam's apple—but not onto it, applying a very hard pressure all the way. Do that four times. A second circular massage starts at the bottom of the ears and ends just below the Adam's apple, alongside the cartilage. Do that four times.

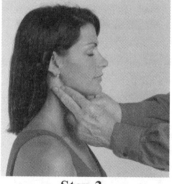

Step 3

4. Stand to the person's left. You're going to work on the back of the head, using your right thumb and middle finger. (On yourself, use both thumbs.) Find the middle of each ear. From there, go straight in toward the medulla oblongata, the hollow at the base of the skull.

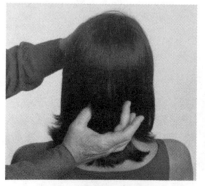

Step 4

5. About 11/2 to 2 inches inward from each ear, there's a lump, a little node. Press these. Move inward half the remaining distance to the medulla on each side, and press. Then place your thumb on the medulla and press.

6. Come down the neck 1/2 inch from the medulla. Place thumb and middle finger on both sides of

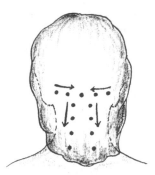

Steps 4,5,6,7

the spinal column, about an inch apart. (On yourself, use both thumbs.) Don't press on the spinal column; press right next to it on both sides simultaneously toward the front of the body.

7.   Press three to five pairs of points, depending on how long the neck is. Go straight down, skipping an inch between points. Stop at the shoulders.

8.   Repeat steps 4 to 7.

Stiff Neck and Sore Shoulders

One of the most common, most annoying complaints I hear from people at my seminars is that they are bothered by stiff necks and shoulders. The type of lifestyle and work behavior that is common now, particularly long periods of sitting in front of a computer or texting on a cell phone, causes us to lean over and crunch up our shoulders. This position causes stiffness.

A number of times I've had to fly a red-eye from the West coast to the East coast. If you've flown, you know the seats only recline down a short distance. Sometimes, I've woken up at the end of the flight with a very stiff neck. I'll do the following treatment on myself so that I can experience immediate relief. While the instructions are written as if you are doing the treatment on a partner, you will find the differences to do on yourself in parenthesis.

Press each point three seconds. The person being treated should sit upright, glasses off, eyes closed, in a comfortable position.

1.   Stand on the left side of the person. Support his/her forehead with your left hand.
2.   You'll be using your right thumb and middle finger, while you are pressing at the back of the head. (When treating yourself, use both thumbs.) First, find the back middle of each ear. From there, move the thumb and finger

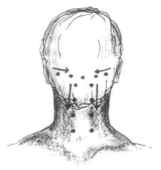

Steps 2 and 3

inward toward each other, on a straight line toward the medulla (the hollow at the base of the skull, just above the neck). About 11/2 to 2 inches from the back of the ears, you'll find a pair of lumps—little nodes. Press these nodes simultaneously with thumb and middle finger. Move half the distance inward toward the medulla on each side, and press again. Then place your thumb in the medulla hollow and press.

3. Move down the neck 1/2 inch from the medulla. Place the thumb and middle finger on both sides of the spinal column, about one inch apart. (On yourself, use both thumbs.) Don't press directly on the spine; press right next to it on both sides. Press three or four pairs of points, depending on how long the neck is. Just go straight down, an inch at a time. Stop at the shoulders.

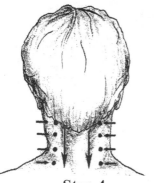

Step 4

4. Go back to 1/2 inch below the medulla. This time place the thumb and middle finger on both sides of the spine, about 2 inches apart. (On yourself, use both thumbs.) This time, press your thumb and finger (or both thumbs) toward each other. Press three or four pairs of points, going down the neck as in Step 4. Stop at the shoulders.

5. Stand directly behind the person. Draw an imaginary line along the top of each shoulder. Using your thumbs, press pairs of points starting at the base of the neck and moving outward an inch at a time, to the top of the arms.

6. (On yourself, treat one shoulder at a time. Place your right middle finger on top of your index fingernail. Bring your right hand across your body as if saluting the flag to the base of your neck. Use the combined pressure of your two fingers to press the points along the top of your shoulder, going outward to your arm. Then use your other arm in the same way to treat the other shoulder.)

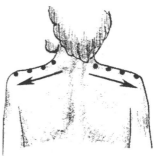

Step 6

7. Repeat the entire process two or three times. (On yourself, repeat it three or four times.)

"Better than a Massage" (Full Back Treatment)

You can't do this treatment on yourself because you can't reach all the points. Besides being a great massage technique, this treatment is excellent for promoting general health and well-being, as it stimulates the entire body.

This massage is unusual in that it is effective even if the person is fully clothed. However, feel free to use full or partial nudity, oils, candles, or whatever you prefer for a more sensuous Shiatsu massage. None of these trimmings is necessary, and all are fine if you'd like to add them.

Have the person lie face down on a firm surface and close his/her eyes. I suggest staying on the left side of the person you're working on. If you straddle the person, don't sit on the buttocks, since this can cause a strain on the person's back.

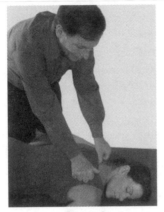

Step 2

1. Do a circular massage between the shoulder blades with the palm of your right hand. Rub with a firm pressure, using fairly rapid movement, and continue for about thirty seconds. Remember to stay between the shoulder blades (not the neck), This part of the back is called the web area, and it contains many nerve endings, so you are affecting and loosening a much larger area than you're actually rubbing.

2. To get an idea of where you'll be pressing, use your thumbs to trace down the spinal column from the top of the shoulder blades to the coccyx, or tailbone. Throughout this treatment, keep your arms straight with the elbows locked. Lean your body weight onto your arms while pressing each point. Never press directly on the spinal column—always on both sides of it. **Press each point three to seven seconds**.

3. Place your thumbs alongside the spine, about an inch apart, at the top of the shoulder blades. Work down from the shoulder blades, skipping an inch between points while pressing along the spine until you get to the tailbone. Use the heel of your hand to apply pressure on the tailbone.

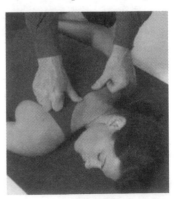

Step 3

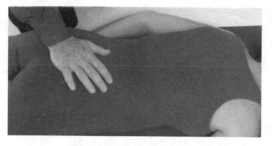

Step 3 Tail Bone Point

4. Find the hips and trace your fingers along the hipbone from your spine to the side of the body. Come back to where the hip and spine meet. Work outward along the hipbone, toward the sides of the body, pressing four evenly spaced points on each side. Press on both sides simultaneously with your thumbs.

5. Return to the place where the spine and hipbone meet. The next four point-pairs form an inverted V, which ends in the middle of each buttock. Press with both thumbs simultaneously.

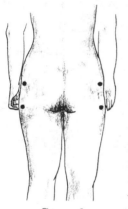

6. Find the upper outer area of the buttocks toward the sides of the body and press down on both sides. Then move to the lower outer part of the buttocks and press.

7. Steps 3 to 6 are done at least twice and possibly three times for one complete treatment or massage.

8. To conclude the massage,

Steps 4-5 Back Points

Step 6

you "chop wood," as if the person's back was a log. Turn your hand sideways, so the fleshy outside of your hand is toward the person's back. Keep your hands slightly cupped and relaxed. Chop rapidly up one side of the person's back and down the other—don't chop directly on top of the spine. Move your hands from your elbows. You can chop pretty hard, and you should hear a good, solid thumping sound. Do this for thirty seconds to a minute.

9. Tell the person to remain still until he/she feels ready to get up.

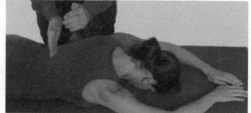

Step 8 "Chopping Wood"

Chapter 4
Exercise and Yoga

Do you think you are too stressed to find time to exercise? Think again. Exercise offers a natural remedy that brings the body into balance when difficult times threaten to throw us out of balance. It is a great stress-reduction strategy, and it works as well—or better—than antidepressants. Sure, when life seems overwhelming—too much to do in too little time—the first thing you may be tempted to skip is your morning workout. But a good daily workout releases hormones into the body that lower your tension and bring a sense of balance to your life.

Exercise counteracts the fight-or-flight response of stress. It can help release feelings of anger, induce a sense of calm, and launch endorphins—the body's "feel good" hormones that have been shown to promote a sense of euphoria. Exercise relieves muscular tension and physical discomfort, improves sleep, and boosts the immune system. It encourages a sense of optimism and hope, enhances self-esteem, and increases energy. A brisk, twenty-minute walk will launch those "feel-good" endorphins and begin to relieve anxiety. You want to exercise around four hours a week for optimal benefits.

It's never too late to start an exercise program. Researchers have found that even people in their 80s can extend their life by exercising as little as four hours a week. Those studied also experienced less depression and loneliness and a greater ability to perform daily tasks.

Do you wonder where you're going to find enough time to work out? New research suggests that even brief bursts of activity can alleviate stress. British researchers studied 20,000 people and found that just twenty minutes a week of moderate activity can significantly reduce the risk of psychological stress. A study by Northern Arizona University researchers claims that just ten minutes of cycling on a stationary bicycle improves energy and mood—even more than a half-hour ride!

Take the first steps to a stress-busting exercise routine: A brisk, midday walk around the office parking lot or a few quick trips up and down a flight of stairs will get you started. And if you take those steps after eating, even for ten or fifteen minutes, it is believed that you can control your insulin and reduce blood sugar spikes to discourage fat storage and reduce the risk of heart disease.

Gentle exercise practices, such as yoga, have also been proven to relieve anxiety. Yoga, has been used for thousands of years to promote a sense of inner peace, relaxation, and well-being.

Hatha Yoga:
Stretching The Body and The Mind

Hatha Yoga is a way of relaxing and stretching your body, which in turn relaxes your mind. As you do these postures (exercises) you'll find yourself becoming more aware of your body and how it feels and functions. I have been doing yoga for 38 years, and do yoga every morning for fifteen to twenty minutes as a way of starting my day.

As you may know; there are many types of yoga. There is a yoga of work (karma), a yoga of love (bakti), a yoga of philosophy (jnana) and others. Some of the teachings and practices are at least 5,000 years old.

Hatha Yoga is the physical yoga, which uses the physical postures or "asanas" as a means of achieving union with the universe. Since yoga is not a religion, it is totally compatible with whatever religious philosophy an individual might be following. Many different styles of yoga have

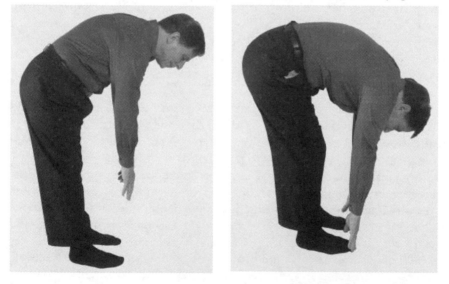

been developed in this country in recent years. I'm going to be focusing on the more traditional Hatha Yoga. You might want to experiment with the different types available in your area to find one that you like the best.

One of the key elements of yoga is that it is non-competitive. You are not competing against an expert, a friend, or even against yourself. This means you don't push yourself further than you can go; don't attempt to push through any pain you are experiencing. Yoga is the opposite of the "no pain, no gain" philosophy. You're just going up to the pain point—the uncomfortable point—and moving back from it so that you stay comfortable.

Hatha Yoga is done very slowly, so that you flow into a position, hold it, and flow out of it. Let your body regulate its own stretches. Some days you stretch more than other days. Stretching in the morning is always harder than later in the day, but morning yoga helps you start the day feeling limber and energetic.

I recommend doing the yoga postures in this book every morning for two weeks. Then, for a pleasant surprise, do it in the afternoon. Since your muscles are looser in the afternoon just from your daily activities, you'll be amazed at the progress you've made. You'll be able to stretch farther than you ever have!

While you can do any of the postures right now, just to relax, for general health I recommend starting with doing one posture a day for a few minutes. At the end of a week, you've put in only 35 minutes and have stretched your body seven different ways. Of course, it's fine to start out with doing more of the postures if you want to, especially if you are in reasonable shape.

Many people conceive of yoga as a series of difficult contortions that takes years of study and practice. That's not necessarily true. It may take quite a while to reach advanced yoga postures that look truly impossible. But it all starts with some very simple movements. The ones I present here are easy, effective, and can be done by anyone. The point is always to stay comfortable when you are stretching. If bending only a few inches is a comfortable stretch for you, that's fine. From doing yoga on a regular basis, you will find yourself stretching farther and farther.

Before I started doing yoga, I had what I would describe as a "bad back." It was frequently annoying me with discomfort, and once every couple of months, my back would "go out," causing me to stand crookedly, limp awkwardly, and feel extreme pain in any position except lying down. At the age of 24, I had lived with this for most of my teen and adult life. When I first tried yoga nearly forty years ago, I couldn't stretch more than a few inches in some directions. The feedback that I receive now at age 62 is a look of disbelief as to how old I am and how young I look and move.

A few other points to keep in mind:

Always do yoga slowly (butterfly and back roll are the only exceptions in this book). *The slower the better.* Imagine it as a drifting, floating, gentle movement into each posture...rather than a bouncing or jerking. During the writing of this book, my collaborator came to me with a complaint. "This umbrella posture (p. 52) is too hard. I can't get anywhere with it! You'll have to change it," she said. I had her try it, and saw that she was moving quickly, as if doing calisthenics. I told her to try it again, much more slowly. Doing the posture at about 1/3 her previous speed, she found it easy.

Although some yoga movements may resemble callisthenic movements, there really is no similarity. The slowness, avoidance of strain and breathing in yoga make it a completely different process and a different experience for the person doing it.

Proper breathing is a very important part of yoga, and breathing instructions are included with each posture. The right breathing makes the postures easier, and allows you to achieve a great feeling of lightness and relaxation. Except where otherwise noted, breathing is done through the nose.

Once you have learned the postures, you will enjoy doing yoga even more with your eyes closed.

Before starting yoga, read the Total Relaxation Pose (next section).

Things to keep in mind:
- If you have a heart problem, you can do yoga with your doctor's permission. When you exercise, just make sure to tense your muscles very gently.
- For women, if it is within three days before your menstrual period, avoid doing the leg raises and back rolls.
- People with lung problems should do the postures very gently.

Total Relaxation Pose

The benefits of yoga are many-faceted. The movements are good for stretching and toning the muscles, gently exercising the heart and lungs, adding to gracefulness, bodily control and general health. However, the relaxation in yoga comes after the movements...during the total relaxation pose, when the muscles relax in response to the stretching and tightening that has just taken place.

Do the Total Relaxation Pose after completing each yoga posture, and for five minutes at the end of your yoga session. Even if you do no other yoga, the total relaxation pose for five minutes a day will help you feel more relaxed and rested.

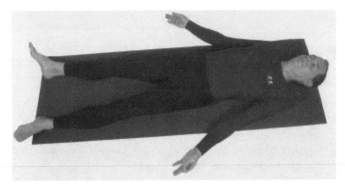

1. Lie down on your back with arms alongside your body, but slightly away from your sides. Turn palms upward. Let your fingers curl so that thumb and index finger form a circle. Your legs should be slightly apart with toes turned outward.
2. The important part of this pose is your breathing. Breathe deeply into your abdomen, filling up your entire stomach. Inhale slowly and exhale slowly through the nostrils. Continue this deep breathing the entire time you are in the position. There is no holding the breath, just moving it slowly in and out.
3. When resting between other postures, don't go on to the next posture until your heart and breath rate have returned to normal. Again, at the end of your yoga session or when doing this by itself, continue for five minutes.
4. When you are finished, turn the palms down and raise your body up slowly.

Neck Exercises

Ours is a society of stiff necks. People spend a lot of time with their necks in one position while working on a computer, talking on a cell phone, texting, reading, studying, or watching television. This exercise will eliminate all soreness and tension.

The entire sequence of movements takes only a couple of minutes, once you know it. It's a good thing to do in the morning while taking a shower with the hot water hitting your neck.

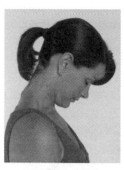

Step 2

Many people tend naturally to stretch their necks in these ways when they feel tense, but they often do it in a fast, jerky manner. This yanks the muscles and is not as relaxing as stretching slowly, gently, and smoothly. A fast movement may feel more effective at first, but that's because the muscles are protesting and holding back. You can actually pull a muscle this way. If you keep up a slow pace from beginning to end, you'll feel how much more relaxed your muscles are.

1. Sit in a chair with your feet flat on the floor. If you are comfortable you can sit in a cross-legged position on the floor. If you wear glasses, take them off. When you get to a hold instruction, keep that position for a second or two. Close your eyes.

2. Drop your chin toward your chest to a slow count of 1...2...3.... Hold for a second or two.

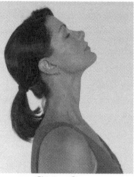

Step 3

3. Begin to raise your head upright, 1...2...3...and continue backward without stopping: 4...5...6... back as far as your head will go without strain. Hold.

4. Slowly repeat steps 2 and 3 two more times. Then bring your head upright again.

5. Slowly drop your left ear toward your left shoulder, 1...2...3... without raising your shoulders. Hold for a second or two. Your head doesn't have to touch your shoulder; if stretching two inches is all that feels comfortable, that's fine.

6. Raise your head upright, 1...2...3... and lower it, 4...5...6... toward your right shoulder. Hold. Then raise your head upright and repeat these sideways stretches twice more. Finally, re-center your head upright.

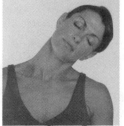

Step 5

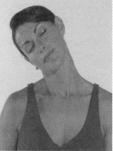

Step 6

7. Without moving your back or shoulders, turn your head as if looking over your left shoulder, 1...2...3...4. Go as far as you comfortably can, and hold it.

8. Turn slowly to the right to a count of eight and look over your right shoulder. Hold it. Repeat

these movements, rotating slowly from side to side twice more. Don't let your shoulders hunch up. You'll be feeling the muscles that connect the neck and shoulders stretching and relaxing.

9. Center your head upright. Drop your chin to your chest and circle your head to the left to a slow count of eight. 1...2...3...4... you're half way around...5...6...7...8...it's a complete circle. Let your head feel like

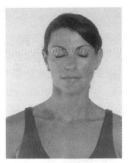

**Step 9
Head Upright**

it's just rolling through the movement. Do two more of these slow circles to the left. Now circle to the right: 1...2...3...4.... 5...6...7...8.... Do it two more times.

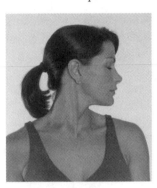

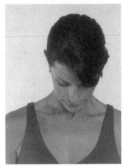

**Step 9
Drop to Chest**

10. Center your head upright. Don't open your eyes. Rub your palms together, building up a lot of friction, which you will feel as heat. Rub them fast, till they feel very hot. With your eyes still closed, place your palms at the back of your neck and inhale through your nose, deeply and slowly. Feel the life-giving energy, the vitality, the heat coming into your neck through your palms. Exhale through your mouth. Feel any tension, any strain, any remaining fatigue going out from your neck through your mouth. Continue inhaling and exhaling at least four times.

11. Relax. Drop your hands. Open your eyes.

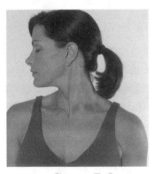

Steps 7-8

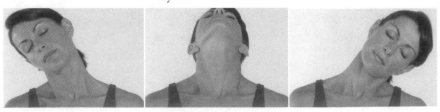

Circle Around Slowly

Eye Exercises

Our eyes are always being bombarded by things to look at–computer screens, cell phone and iPod screens, billboards, signs, movies, TV, and the things we read for work, study, or pleasure. Our eyes are so active that we may develop eyestrain without knowing it. This makes us feel tired, headachy, or unable to concentrate, when it's really just our eyes that need a rest.

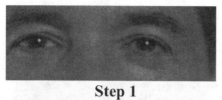

Step 1

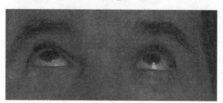

Step 2

Practice these exercises two or three times with your eyes open, so you know how it feels when you are moving your eyes in the right direction. After you know the movements, the entire sequence should be done without opening the eyes. You will find it more relaxing that way.

1. Sitting upright, focus on a point directly in front of you as your center point. (When you do this with your eyes closed, it will be an imaginary point.)

2. Without moving your head, raise your eyes up toward the ceiling, as high as they can go without straining. Only move your eyes, nothing else. Hold for a few seconds.

3. Move your eyes toward the floor as far as they can go. Hold for a few seconds.

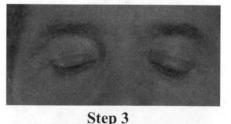

Step 3

4. Repeat the upward and downward movements twice more. Always hold for a second or two at the farthest points. Bring the eyes back to center and gaze ahead of you for a few moments.

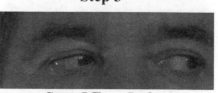

Step 5 Eyes Left

5. Move your eyes to the left as far as you can go comfortably. Hold. Then move your eyes all the way to the right as far as you can and hold. Repeat this twice more. Bring the eyes back to the center and gaze ahead of you for a few moments.

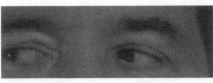

Step 5 Eyes Right

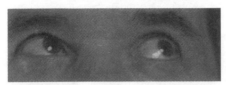

Step 6 Diagonally Up Left

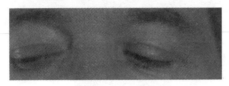

Step 6 Diagonally Down Right

6. Move your eyes diagonally up to the left. Hold. Then diagonally down to the right. Hold. Do this twice more. Center and gaze.

7. Move your eyes diagonally up to the right—hold—then diagonally down to the left—hold. Repeat twice more. Return to the center point and gaze.

8. Now make complete circles slowly with your eyes. Don't rush through them. Keep the eyes moving smoothly and don't stop and hold at any point. Begin by moving your eyes left, then down, then to the right, then up, then left again. Circle to the left twice more. Return to the center point and gaze a few seconds.

9. Now circle to the right, down, to the left, up, and to the right again. Continue through two more circles to the right. Come back to the center and gaze.

10. Keeping your eyes closed, rub your palms together, building up a lot of friction, a lot of heat. Rub them fast. When the palms feel very hot, place them over your eyes—just cupping your palms over your eyes, not pressing on them. Inhale very deeply and slowly. Feel energy, vitality and heat coming from your palms into

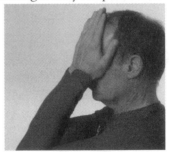

Step 10

your eyes. Exhale rapidly through your mouth, and feel yourself exhaling any remaining strain or fatigue that may be in your eyes. Continue inhaling and exhaling at least three or four times.

11. Relax. (Ah...) This exercise feels much better with the eyes closed than open. If it's hard for you to believe that your eyes are moving properly when closed, do this: Close them and gently place your fingertips on the eyelids. Now move your eyes to either side. Hold. You will feel the movement so that you will know that you've done the movement correctly.

The Butterfly

The Butterfly stretches the inner thigh and relaxes the legs. It's a great warm-up and unwinding exercise to do before and after sports. Use it to limber up for swimming, gymnastics, tennis, bike riding, climbing, and hiking.

If your legs are stiff from some activity, or from standing on your feet all day, this simple movement will relax them, When you stand, your legs have to work against gravity, sending waste-carrying blood "uphill" to the heart. The Butterfly makes this easier by stretching and strengthening the leg muscles, increasing circulation.

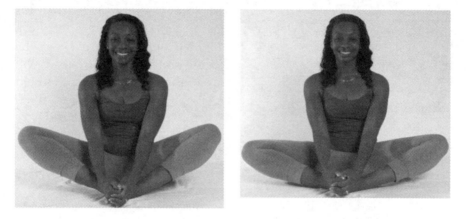

This posture is also recommended as a warm-up for the back roll (see the next posture).

1. Sitting on the floor, bring the soles of your feet together, as close to your body as is comfortable, so that you look like you have wings.
2. Hold onto your toes with your hands, keep your back straight, and flap your legs up and down as if you were flying. The sides of your feet should stay on the floor while your knees go up and down.

FLAP AT A RAPID RATE—this is one yoga posture that is not done slowly. As you are flapping, put a slight pulling pressure on your feet, pulling them toward your body. Flap for at least thirty seconds.

Back Roll

This warm-up exercise for yoga will stretch the spinal column and lengthen and relax the back muscles. Most people don't exercise their backs much, although they do put strain on their backs, sitting in office chairs staring at a computer monitor, sitting in a car, sitting at a school desk and the like. So this exercise is good for almost anyone.

1. Sit on the floor with your knees drawn up to your chest and feet flat on the floor. Knees can be apart. Clasp your forearms just under your knees. The proper breathing in this exercise is to exhale while rolling backward, inhale while rolling forward.

2. Roll backward as far as you can, stretching your legs out as you go. If you can, attempt to have your toes touch the floor behind your head. After you have gone back that far, roll forward to your starting position. If you can't roll back so that your toes touch the floor, just rock back and forth on your spine as far as comfortable.

You don't have to do this exercise slowly, and you don't hold at any one point. Just roll back and forth, six to fifteen times. You can even roll on the area to the left of the spinal column and then to the right. This will stretch and exercise an even larger area of the back.

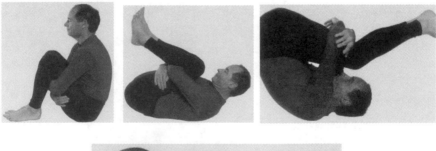

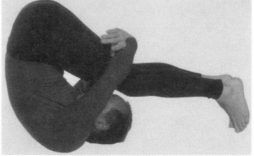

Leg Raises

Leg Raises are excellent for strengthening the legs and stomach muscles while warming up the body for doing other postures.

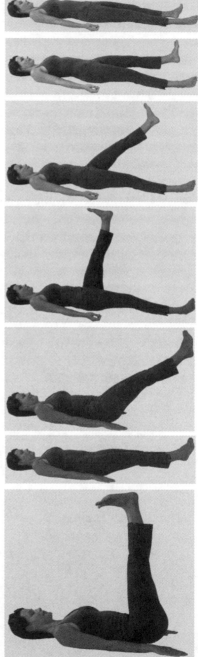

1. Lie on your back, hands at your sides with palms down
2. Raise your left leg...first six inches...then twelve inches...then straight up to form a ninety-degree angle to the floor. Do this as slowly as you can manage. (But remember, if you feel pain, don't stretch any further.) Always keep your leg straight, even if this means you can't raise it as far as you'd like.
3. Lower slowly your leg to the floor.
4. Raise and lower your left leg three times. Repeat with your right leg...six inches... then twelve inches...then straight up. Lower slowly each time.
5. Raise both legs together... six inches off the floor... twelve inches...then straight up. (This will be harder at first than raising each leg separately. The most important thing is to keep legs straight.) Lower slowly back down. Do this three times.
6. Do the Total Relaxation Pose (p. 42).

The Cat Bow

The Cat Bow stretches the spine and the chest, relieves neck strain, and helps firm the stomach muscles.

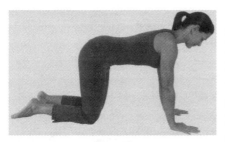

Step 1

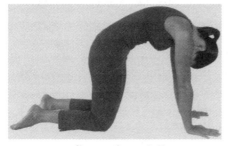

Steps 3 and 5

1. Take a position on your hands and knees as if you were a cat. Place hands about shoulder-width apart.

2. Inhale deeply and slowly through your nose, filling your stomach and chest.

3. While exhaling, lower your head and bring your chin to your chest, and curve your back upward toward the ceiling. Hold that pose, with empty lungs.

4. As you begin to inhale, turn your fingers inward, so that they are facing each other. Raise your head up. Lower your chest toward the floor between your fingertips, bending your elbows. Go down as far as is comfortable and hold that position with lungs full. Hold for several seconds.

5. Begin to exhale, turning your fingers outward again. Bring your chin to your chest while you straighten your arms and curve your back upward. Hold with empty lungs for several seconds.

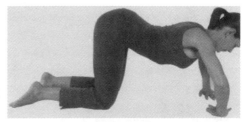

Step 4. Lowering

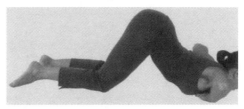

Step 4. Fully Lowered

6. Do these movements four to six times, at a slow pace. Remember to stay comfortable.

7. Do the Total Relaxation Pose (p. 42).

Umbrella

Excellent for the stomach, backs of the legs, and the upper and lower back.

1. Place your feet a little less than shoulder width apart. Place your arms behind your back and intertwine your fingers. Pull your shoulders back. Inhale.
2. As you exhale, bend from the waist toward your left leg, keeping your back arched, head up. While bending, raise your arms up toward the ceiling, raising them up behind you as far as you can comfortably go. Hold for a few seconds at your furthest point. While bending, keep your back arched and head up as long as possible, then try to touch your forehead to your knee. (If you can't do this, just bend as far as you can comfortably.)
3. While inhaling…raise your head, arch your back and lower arms. Meanwhile, slowly return to the starting position.
4. Repeat the same bending and raising movements toward your right leg Each time you've gone down and up once, you can take a few breaths to rest before continuing. Do this exercise three times in each direction.
5. Finish with the Total Relaxation Pose (p. 42).

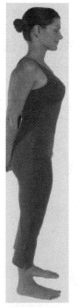 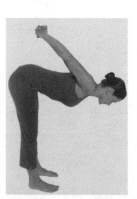 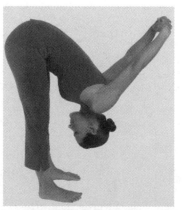

Step 1   **Step 2. Lowering**   **Step 2. Fully Lowered**

Posterior Stretch

This posture may feel difficult at first, since most of us in this society are sitting-oriented. Unless we're active hikers, ballet dancers, or tennis players, we don't get much stretching of the hamstring muscles which are located at the back of the leg). When you begin doing Posterior Stretch, don't be surprised if you can initially move only a few inches. (That was about the farthest I could move before I began doing yoga regularly… remember the pictures on page 40.) By the end of two weeks, you'll be amazed at how far you can stretch.

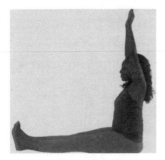

Steps 1-2

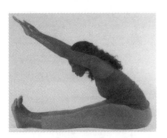

Step 3. Lowering

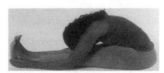

**Step 3.
Fully Lowered**

1.   Sit on the floor, legs straight out in front of you, feet together. Your weight should be on the front portion of your buttocks, almost on your thighs. To get there, imagine that you are walking, taking four steps forward. Go through that motion. Sit erect.

2.   As you inhale, slowly raise your arms along the sides of your body, stretching toward the ceiling. With arms up as far as they can go, hold the stretch for a second or two.

3.   Keeping your back arched and your head up, lower your upper body toward your legs. Move slowly. Always keep your legs straight. When you have lowered yourself as far as you can go, hold onto the part of the leg that is closest to your hand. Hold for two or three seconds, keeping your lungs empty. (If you can touch your chin to your legs and grasp your toes, you are way beyond the beginner stage.)

4.   Begin to inhale and move upward again with your arms still stretched in front of you and your back arched.

5.   When you are straight up again, slowly lower your arms to your lap and exhale.

6.   Rest until breathing and heartbeat are back to normal before doing this two more times. If you like, you can put your hands on the floor by your sides for support while resting.

7.   Finish with the Total Relaxation Pose (p. 42).

The Cobra

The Cobra tones and strengthens and stretches the back and stomach muscles. It can aid in the prevention of lower back problems and pain.

1. Lie on your stomach, feet together. Place your palms on the floor beside your shoulders, with fingers forward. Your forehead should be on the floor. Inhale.

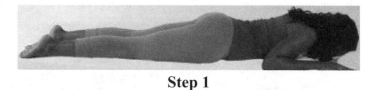

Step 1

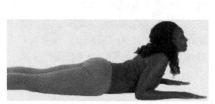

Step 2. Raising

2. While exhaling, slowly lift your head up and back as far as comfortable. Then, without using your arms, lift your shoulders and chest. When you cannot lift any further, begin to use your arms to raise yourself even further up, keeping your head back and your back arched. You must keep your hips and stomach on the floor, which means you may not be able to straighten your arms completely. Hold with lungs empty at the highest point you can reach without raising your hips and stomach off the floor.

3. Begin to inhale. Lower slowly by easing down first onto your stomach... then chest...then forehead.

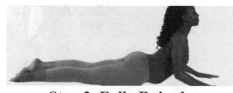

Step 2. Fully Raised

4. Bring your hands up to form a pillow under your forehead. Rest until your breathing and heartbeat return to normal. Repeat the exercise twice more.

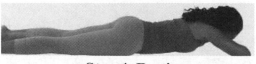

Step 4. Resting

5. After the third repetition, return to the Total Relaxation Pose (p. 42).

Chapter 5
Relaxation and Insomnia Relief

Progressive Relaxation

You can do this exercise lying down or sitting upright. If you do it lying down, you're apt to fall asleep, which makes this exercise good for insomnia or temporary sleep difficulty. If you don't fall asleep the first time, do it a second or third time through.

If you do this exercise sitting up, you'll be totally relaxed. It's nice to have someone read the instructions to you, at least the first time through. The reader should read slowly and pause a few seconds between steps. You, or someone whose voice you like, can also put this on an iPod or mp3 player. Be sure to read slowly, and leave pauses for doing each step in the process.

1. If you are lying down, lie on your back with your arms alongside your body, but slightly away from your sides. Turn your palms upward. Let your fingers curl so that thumb and index finger form a circle. Your legs should be slightly apart with toes turned outward. If you are sitting up, put your feet flat on the floor and sit with your spine straight but not stiff. Close your eyes.

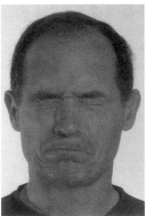

Step 2

2. Tighten your face muscles by squinting your eyes, wrinkling your nose, and tightening all the facial muscles. Keep tightening those muscles...tight...tight...tighter...really tense...tenser...then relax them completely.

3. Inhale very deeply and slowly through your nostrils. Then exhale very deeply and slowly. Feel the tension and strain flowing out of your face.

4. Take your awareness to your neck and shoulders. Tighten them up...really tight...tighter...tense...tense...tenser...then relax them completely.

5. Become aware of your arms. Make a fist and tighten all the muscles in your arms. Tense up your hands, palms, forearms, and triceps. Tighten them...tighter...tighter...even tighter...then relax. Let your hand and arms go completely limp in your lap or by the sides of your body.

6. Inhale and exhale very deeply and slowly through your nostrils. Feel the tension and strain flowing away.

7. Take your awareness to your chest. Tighten all your chest muscles really tight...really tense...tighter...tenser...even tighter...then relax completely.

8. Become aware of your stomach and buttocks. Tighten all of the muscles in your stomach and buttocks really tight...tight...tight...tighter...even tighter...then relax.

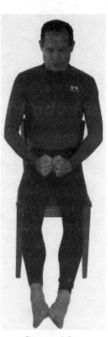

Step 12

9. Inhale very deeply and slowly...and exhale very deeply and slowly.

10. Take your awareness to your legs. Stretch them out in front of you. Arch your toes and tighten all the muscles in your legs...your thighs, your calves, your feet...really tight...tighter...tense...tenser...even tenser...then relax. Feel your legs sinking into the floor...deeper and deeper, as you become more and more relaxed.

11. Inhale and exhale very deeply and slowly.

12. Take your awareness from the very tip of your head to the very bottoms of your feet. Tighten your entire body...make a face...curl your hands...arch your toes...tense your arms...chest...stomach...buttocks...legs...face...tighter...tighter...even tighter...then relax completely.

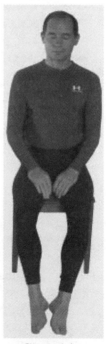

Step 14

13. Inhale very deeply and slowly through the nostrils…exhale very deeply and slowly. Again, inhale and exhale very deeply and slowly.
14. Relax for a few minutes in this position, breathing normally.

Mind and Body Relaxation

This exercise is excellent for recurring insomnia or temporary sleep difficulties, as well as general relaxation and relief of tensions.

In this exercise, you will not be moving at all. You will not even be tensing or contracting your muscles. Instead, you will be telling your body to relax, part by part. By thinking relaxation to your muscles, you can actually get them to relax. This has been demonstrated in experiments with biofeedback, in which people learn to control their heart rate, blood pressure, and brainwave activity just by thinking about what they want those functions to do.

Have someone read this exercise to you, at least the first time, so that you can concentrate on relaxing, not on the reading. It should be read slowly, with a two- to three-second pause after each numbered step. The words in parentheses are instructions to the person doing the reading and should not be read aloud.

If you want, you can record the instructions on an iPod or mp3 player.

1. Lie down on your back in the position described in step one of Progressive Relaxation, page 55. Close your eyes. Become aware of the top of your head. Silently, tell all the muscles in your head to relax. Say to yourself, over and over:

Relaxation Message
"Relax…relax…you are relaxing…you are unwinding…letting all tension flow away…relax…you are letting go of all strain… relaxing…you are relaxing…"
(You can vary the words and add other relaxing words if you wish.)

2. Visualize your muscles completely relaxing, stretching out into a soft, comfortable position like a cat going to sleep.
3. Take your awareness to your forehead. Tell all the muscles in your forehead to relax. Tell the muscles in your forehead to relax by repeating the relaxation message.

4. Take your awareness to your eyes. Tell all the muscles in your eyes to relax. You are not moving your eyes at all; you are just thinking relaxation to them. Tell the eye muscles to relax by repeating the relaxation message.

5. Keep visualizing the relaxation taking place. In your mind you can see all the muscles around your eyes relaxing…and all tension flowing away.

6. Inhale and exhale through your nostrils, very deeply and slowly. Fill your entire stomach and chest with the breath before letting it out, slowly through the nostrils.

7. Take your awareness to your neck. Tell all the muscles in your neck to relax by repeating the relaxation message.

8. Take your awareness to your shoulders. Tell all your shoulder muscles to relax by repeating the relaxation message.

9. Take your awareness to your upper arm. Tell all those muscles to relax. Take your awareness to your forearms. Tell all those muscles to relax. Take your awareness to your hands and fingers. Tell all the muscles in your hands and fingers to completely relax. Visualize the relaxation taking place in your arms, as you tell all of those muscles to relax by repeating the relaxation message.

10. Take your awareness to your fingertips and palms. Feel a tingling sensation in your palms and fingertips. Draw that tingling energy into your body and slowly up your arms. Bring the energy through your forearms…triceps…shoulders… neck. You're still not moving at all. Place the energy at the base of your skull. Tell it to wait there and you'll be back shortly.

11. Inhale and exhale through your nose, very deeply and slowly. Fill your entire stomach and chest with the breath before letting it out, slowly.

12. Now, take your awareness to your chest. Tell all the muscles in your chest to relax. Say to your chest muscles:

Relaxation Message
"Relax…relax…you are relaxing…all tension is draining away…all tightness is flowing out of you…relax…relax…you are relaxing… all tension is melting away…you are completely relaxing…"
(Reader can add or substitute similar words and phrases.)

13. Take your awareness to your stomach. Tell all of your stomach muscles to relax by repeating the relaxation message.

14. Take your awareness to your buttocks. Tell every muscle in your buttocks to relax by repeating the relaxation message.

15. Inhale very slowly and deeply, through your nose, filling your stomach and chest. Exhale slowly through your nose.

16. Take your awareness to your thighs. Tell all the muscles in your thighs to relax. Take your awareness to your calves. Tell all the muscles in your calves to relax. Take your awareness to your feet and toes. Tell all the muscles in your feet and toes to relax. Visualize all the muscles in your legs relaxing and unwinding, visualize all tension leaving as you repeat the relaxation message to every one of your leg muscles.

17. Take your awareness to the bottoms of your feet. Feel a tingling sensation. Begin to draw that energy into your body, up to your mind. Draw the energy slowly through your feet, ankles...calves...thighs...buttocks. Place that energy at the base of your spine. Then move it slowly up the spine to right below the navel...then to the abdomen...then the heart... then the throat. Have that energy join with the energy from your arms that you left at the base of your skull. Let all that energy enter your mind and place it at the point between your eyebrows. Hold it there for a few seconds...then quickly release all the energy back through your entire body, letting it rush out through your arms and legs. When you are finished, just stay still and enjoy the feelings of relaxation.

Chapter 6
Meditation

Meditation is absolutely amazing. It can totally revitalize your entire system in a very, very short period of time. Research on the physiology of meditation has shown that it slows the heart rate by about five beats per minute. Breath rate slows down. All the vital signs—blood pressure, muscle tension, etc.—are greatly slowed. Meditation has even cured high blood pressure. Meditation will also slow down the aging process as measured by a person's vital signs by ten years in a long-term meditator.

During meditation, your brain produces an abundance of alpha waves, described as a state of relaxed awareness. As a matter of fact, meditation produces a lower rate of body activity than is reached even in the deepest part of sleep. This is why twenty minutes of meditation gives you as much deep rest and rejuvenation as six to eight hours of sleep.

Most people who meditate regularly find they need less sleep. I used to need nine to ten hours a night, but now with meditation I need only six and a half to seven hours. Meditating regularly takes just fifteen to twenty minutes twice a day. So, you gain time in your day by needing less sleep and by having more energy, which means you can get more done.

When I first started to meditate, I thought I would have to give up thirty to forty minutes a day. I was surprised when I realized I had actually gained several hours a day of time to be active getting things done. Now I am even able to undergo dental procedures without painkillers and hernia surgery with only a local anesthesia. Even my doctors are amazed!

Do you wake up in the morning with the world groggy and your eyes fuzzy and an urge to throw

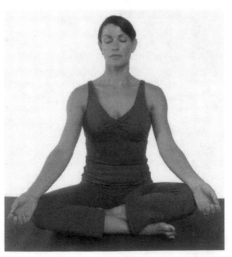

the alarm clock out the window? I did. After your morning meditation, you'll be clear-headed and raring to go, which as I said is what happened to me

After a day of work, study or play, your early evening meditation will refresh your body and mind. Instead of wanting to crawl into bed and go to sleep, you'll feel wide awake and ready to go again.

Meditation can make life easier for persons whose jobs sometimes require them to do without sleep, such as reporters, medical personnel, firefighters, military personnel, and computer programmers. If you are working on an all-night project or studying for an exam, meditate once more at midnight. This will enable you to stay awake. When morning comes and your head is spinning, do your regular morning meditation. You'll be alert and ready for the day. (Note: This third meditation should be done only occasionally, not daily.)

Speaking of sleep, many people ask. "What's to keep me from falling sleep while I meditate?" Nothing, but don't worry about it because falling asleep is a natural part of the meditation process. Your body is saying, "Wow, you are giving me this opportunity to rest and I'm taking it. I'm tired." When you wake up and realize you've been sleeping, don't open your eyes immediately and get up. Instead take an extra five minutes of meditation time; otherwise you may not feel completely refreshed.

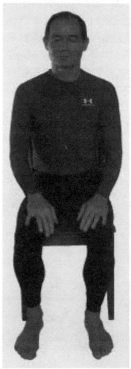

Falling asleep is actually a deeper level of relaxation for the body. Since you are already in a state that is deeper than the deepest state of sleep, you are giving your body a tremendous amount of rest and relaxation when you fall into a mediation-type of sleep. I use the term "mediation-type sleep" on purpose. Normally when you fall asleep and someone or something wakes you up, initially you are groggy and have difficulty clearing your mind and functioning. When you are in a meditative-type sleep and you hear someone or something, you are instantly back at an effective, functioning level. While falling asleep is not the purpose of meditation, it is an important part of the process.

To avoid deliberately falling asleep, you want to do the mediation sitting in a chair or in a comfortable cross-legged position on the floor.

Another interesting fact about meditation is that you don't really need quiet and solitude for it. It might feel better in a quiet place, but research indicates this isn't necessary.

This was discovered when scientists tested meditators with instruments that measure certain vital signs, such as heartbeat, brainwaves, and breath rate. After the meditation the researchers asked, "How did it feel?" Some subjects said, "Great, best meditation I've ever had." Others said it was terrible: They hardly could sit still; they were distracted by the machines; they couldn't concentrate on relaxing. But the readings of their vital signs showed that all subjects were at the same deep levels of rest and relaxation. These results indicate that no matter how you feel about your meditation, you're doing fine as long as you sit there and do it for the required time.

This also means that you can meditate in a car, a plane, and even a cafeteria or anywhere you need to do it. It may not feel like the best meditation you've ever had, but it's still working.

As long as three decades ago, researchers in this country were proving the benefits of meditation. Among their findings:

- Meditators can withstand more life changes with less illness than non-meditators.
- Meditation develops the ability to solve life problems, and to cope with feelings of hopelessness and depression.
- Experienced meditators feel more in control of their lives than beginning meditators.
- Meditators report feeling much less anxiety each day than non-meditators.
- Meditators have fewer colds, headaches, and sleeping difficulties.
- Meditators react faster to a tension-producing event, both physically and mentally, than non-meditators. After the event is over, meditators relax quickly and easily. Non-meditators stay tense much longer. (Some didn't relax at all during the research time.)
- Meditation trains the capacity to pay attention.

Transcendental Meditation is perhaps the best-known method of meditation, thanks to the Beetles, who made it a household topic in the 1960s. It is also one of the most thoroughly researched. More than 600 scientific studies have been conducted over the last forty years, verifying the following benefits of Transcendental Meditation:

- Greater orderliness of brain functioning
- Improved ability to focus
- Increased creativity
- Deeper level of relaxation
- Improved perception and memory
- Increased development of intelligence
- Decrease in stress hormone
- Lower blood pressure
- Reversal of the aging process
- Reduced need for medical care
- Reduction in cholesterol
- Increased self-actualization
- Increased strength of self-concept
- Decreased cigarette, alcohol, and drug abuse
- Increased productivity
- Improved relations at work

Regular meditators consistently report that they are happier, more at ease with themselves, and better able to cope with personal problems than before they began meditating.

When I first heard these kinds of statements years ago I said, "Hah! That couldn't be." I was extremely skeptical. Nothing that simple could cause such enormous changes in one's life. However, I looked at the early physiological studies that had been done on meditation, which indicated that at least I might get some energy from it. So I tried it. After I'd been meditating for a while, I asked some close friends if, quite honestly, they had noticed any changes in me. They told me that I seemed happier, more joyous, and more at ease with myself. It was like hearing a recording of what I'd been told would happen. I suggest that you meditate regularly for at least two or three weeks so you can make your own determination of the benefits from meditation that you are experiencing.

Do's and Don'ts of Meditation

THE KEY TO GETTING ALL THE BENEFITS FROM MEDITATION IS TO MEDITATE REGULARLY, TWICE A DAY, FOR FIFTEEN TO TWENTY MINUTES EACH TIME. In the morning, do it anytime before breakfast. If you don't eat breakfast, do it before you start your day's activities. In the late afternoon, do it anytime before dinner.

You can also substitute several shorter meditation periods of 5 to 10 minutes at a time throughout the day. So long as the minutes total thirty to forty minutes, you'll get the benefits.

1. GIVE IT A CHANCE TO WORK. During the first two weeks, stay away from any drugs, medication, or alcohol. This will give you a chance to distinguish the changes that are happening just from meditating.

2. IF YOU WEAR CONTACT LENSES, REMOVE THEM. Otherwise, you may wind up meditating on the pain in your eyes.

3. IF YOU FIND YOURSELF THINKING OF OTHER THINGS, DON'T WORRY ABOUT IT. DON'T FIGHT IT. OBSERVE THE THOUGHT, LET IT GO, AND RETURN TO THE MEDITATION TECHNIQUE. Suppose you are meditating, and then you start thinking, "Wonder what I'll have for dinner?" Then you become aware that you've been thinking, not meditating. "Oh, no!" you might think. "I blew it! I'm supposed to make my mind go blank" This is not the right way to react to your thoughts. Don't become angry or upset at yourself and think that you've blow it, because you have not.

   Here's the right way to handle a thought: As you become aware that you've been thinking about what's for dinner, you calmly say to yourself, "Oh, there's a thought." Then you let the thought go without becoming angry with yourself and you simply return to the technique.

4. IF YOU FIND YOUR NECK HURTS WHEN YOU ARE FINISHED MEDIATATING, THEN YOUR HEAD MAY BE DROPPING FORWARD. I have experienced this to the point where I was getting chronic neck pain. I came up with the idea of using a foam neck brace to give me the support I needed. If you begin to have neck pain, you can purchase

a brace at a medical supply store. I've actually worn it when I have had to meditate on planes, and no one has even commented on it. (It is also great for napping on planes— better than those neck wraps that still allow your head to fall forward.)

Possible Intrusions or Distractions:
Worrying
Remembering a fight you had with someone
Daydreaming about someone you love
Unmade decisions
Scenes from a movie you saw last night
Unexpected strong feelings
Things you have to get done
Remembering a Twitter message you should not have sent

What to Do:
1. Observe that the thought is there.
2. Let it go, gently. Don't worry about it or about how it is affecting your meditation.
3. Return to doing the technique you have selected to do.
5. IF YOU HAVE AN ITCH, SCRATCH IT, IMMEDIATELY. If you have to blow your nose, blow it. If your leg falls asleep, move it. If you don't take care of your physical discomforts, you'll end up meditating on them. It is so much easier to just scratch the itch and let it go.
6. IF YOU HAVE TO GET UP WHILE MEDITATING—to answer the phone or the door—THAT'S OKAY. Get up and take care of the interruption, then come back as soon as you can, even if you were almost done, and meditate for another five minutes. While meditating, you've been in a very deep state of physiological rest, and having to get up to handle the disturbance brings you back too suddenly to the waking state. It's a slight shock to your system, so you simply return to meditating for another five minutes to come out of it slowly and smoothly.
7. DON'T MEDITATE JUST BEFORE BEDTIME. It may keep you awake!
8. USE A CLOCK SO YOU CAN KEEP TRACK OF THE MEDITATION TIME PERIOD. While you can attempt to set your own internal biological clock that wakes you up at

7:30 a.m. even on Saturday and Sunday, I'd suggest instead that you have a clock easily in view, so you can open one eye and briefly glance at the time. Don't use an alarm clock to indicate the end of your meditation; it's as jolting as a phone or doorbell ringing.

When you meditate there is a time distortion that usually takes place. The fifteen to twenty minutes may seem to last forever or to go by in a flash, which makes it difficult to set your internal clock accurately. These time distortions will continue to occur, no matter how long you've been practicing meditation.

9. DON'T MEDITATE AFTER EATING. You will wind up meditating on your stomach! A stomach full of food wants to focus on digesting it, so your body will divert extra blood to the stomach. Since meditating reduces your circulation and heart rate, you will experience two systems working in opposite ways—one wanting to speed up, the other wanting to slow down. The conflict will make you mainly aware of your stomach.

10. IF YOU DON'T FEEL RELAXED AND ENERGIZED AFTER OPENING YOUR EYES, MEDITATE FOR ANOTHER FIVE MINUTES. You may have come out of meditating too quickly or not taken the extra five minutes after falling asleep. In that case, another five minutes and "Finishing Up" (p. 72) will have you feeling relaxed and energized again.

11. "HOW DO I KNOW I'M DOING IT RIGHT?" Meditation is a very subjective process. Some meditations you will never want to end, and others you'll feel you hardly want to continue. As I mentioned before, the benefits in your daily life are the same either way. Remember, it works because you do it regularly twice a day.

And Now It's Time to Start

Read this section all the way through before beginning. I've given you a choice of six meditation techniques to experience. If possible, have a friend read two of them to you the first time you meditate. The reader should read one technique and pause while you do it for ten minutes. Then, he or she should softly read another technique to you and pause while you do that one for ten minutes. You should keep your eyes closed the entire time.

If you don't have a friend who can do this, simply read one technique and do it for the full fifteen to twenty minutes. The next time you meditate do another one.

Once you pick a technique that feels comfortable to you, stick to it and continue to do that technique for the first two to three weeks, just so you become even more comfortable with that technique. Then you can experiment with others, if you wish. Stick to any technique you do for at least two to three weeks.

If you are visually oriented, I suggested the Object of Beauty technique; otherwise, you can pick one of the other techniques. There is also a meditation technique for couples that is included in this chapter.

No matter what technique you use, start with the following two instructions, and end with the Finishing Up instruction at the end of this chapter.

- Sit on the floor or in a chair, whichever is more comfortable for you. If you're on the floor, you can cross your legs. In a chair, either cross your legs or place your feet flat on the floor. Hold your spine straight. If you are not accustomed to sitting upright, it's good to have your back supported by a wall or the back of the chair. Otherwise, you'll meditate on the tensions in your back.
- If you have glasses on, take them off. If you have a tight belt, loosen it. If your clothing is constricting, loosen it. Do anything you need to feel unconfined and relaxed.
- Do this exercise to straighten your spine: Raise your arms up over your head and stretch towards the ceiling.

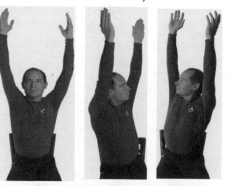

Stretching Your Spine

Stretch your arms and neck up...get a good stretch. Twist your entire body from the waist, first to the left, hold...then to the right, hold. Keep stretching upward throughout the twists. Do the twists slowly. Come back to the center, stretch up one last time, and lower your arms slowly. (See illustration) Your back, which may have felt like a winding country road, is now a highway to send messages of relaxation all over your body.

Hong Saw

1. Keeping your eyes closed, become aware of your breathing. Become aware of your inhalation and exhalation, but don't try to regulate it. Just let your breath do what it wants to do.

2. Now, each time you inhale, you're going to say to yourself, silently, the word "hong." Envision the word entering your head at the point between your eyebrows. (If you can't see the word clearly, it's okay to imagine just the feeling of it entering between your eyebrows.)

3. Each time you exhale, you're going to say silently to yourself the word "saw," and see the word (or the feeling) exiting at the point between your eyebrows.

4. You'll be inhaling and seeing "hong" entering between the eyebrows, then exhaling and seeing "saw" exiting. Remember: just let your saying or feeling the words follow your natural rate of breathing. If your breath becomes shallow, that's fine; if it's deep, that's fine. If it stops, don't worry; you will start breathing again. Don't change your breathing deliberately. Just keep doing "HONG...SAW" for fifteen to twenty minutes.

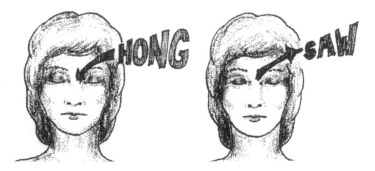

Object of Beauty

1. Find an object, sound, color, word, scene…something that you feel is beautiful to you.
2. Imagine taking that object, sound, color, word, scene, or other beautiful thing and place it at the point between your eyebrows.
3. Examine it there.
4. Gradually, you'll begin to get a feeling of beauty from your object of beauty. Let this feeling fill your entire body.
5. Send this feeling of beauty out and fill the entire room with it. Send the feeling out as far as you're comfortable…to surround the building…the town…and the earth. Even send it into the universe.

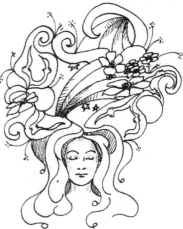

6. If you lose your feeling of beauty, just return to your object of beauty, and reexamine it between your eyebrows until the feeling returns. Then again extend the feeling of beauty outward.
7. Do your best to focus on only one object during each meditation. Continue this technique for fifteen to twenty minutes.

Watching the Breath

1. Close your eyes and begin by becoming aware of your breathing. Don't try and regulate it, just allow the breath to go at whatever rate it wants to go. Simply be aware of what your breath is doing.
2. On your inhalation, feel the coolness of the air coming in through your nose. Follow this coolness as far back into your body as you can.
3. On your exhalation, follow the warmth of the air from as far back in your body as you can comfortably.
4. Just continue to follow the coolness when you inhale and the warmth when you exhale. Continue for fifteen to twenty minutes.

Passage Meditation

In passage meditation, as taught by the Blue Mountain Center of Meditation, you choose a spiritual text or passage that embodies your highest ideals, memorize it, and then repeat the words slowly, silently, and with as much concentration as possible.

1. Close your eyes and begin to go slowly, in your mind, through the words of a simple, positive inspirational passage from one of the world's great spiritual traditions.
2. While meditating, if you begin to think other thoughts about the meaning of the words, simply return to the words themselves. If you are giving your full attention to each word, the meaning will begin to become clear to you.
3. When you reach the end of the passage, you can repeat the passage again from the beginning until you have completed your fifteen to twenty minutes

You can memorize other passages so you can vary which one you use.

Mindfulness Meditation

Jon Kabat-Zinn, Ph.D., a pioneer in the use of mindfulness meditation to treat chronic pain and illness in medical environments, teaches what he calls the Body Scan meditation technique. This technique develops attention and may also be used to still the mind as a prelude to any of the other techniques of meditation, or it can be done by itself. It is similar to the Mind and Body Relaxation exercise on page 57. This is also the only technique done lying down.

1. Lie flat on your back, arms at your sides, palms facing upward. Place a pillow under your knees to alleviate any back pain. Feel your breath, moving in and out of your body. Try to maintain an awareness of the breath while you are scanning the body.
2. Bring your attention to the toes of your left foot, without wiggling them, then to the arch and the heel. Feel the contact with the floor. Move your attention to the ankle, then the calf, and slowly up the leg to the pelvis.
3. Then do the same with your right leg, moving your attention slowly from your toes to the pelvis.
4. Very slowly, move your attention up the torso, through the lower back and abdomen, then to the upper back, the chest,

and the shoulders. Then bring your attention to the fingers on both hands, and move up the arms to the shoulders. Then move through the neck and throat, the face and the back of the head, and then right on up through the top of the head.

5. Relax until you have completed your fifteen to twenty minutes.

Dyadic Meditation or Meditation for Couples

You do this technique with a partner. This meditation is done with your eyes open.

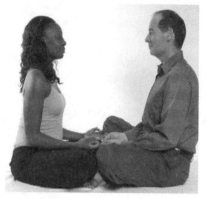

1. Sit opposite each other with knees touching. You can be in two chairs or sitting cross-legged on the floor.
2. Begin looking into your partner's left eye with both your eyes. Your partner will be looking with both eyes into your left eye. If you need to blink, that's okay, but attempt to keep it to a minimum.
3. Do this for fifteen to twenty minutes.
4. When the time is up, gently break eye contact and discuss with your partner what you both felt and experienced.

Finishing Up

After your fifteen to twenty minutes are up, stop doing the technique. Keep your eyes closed. Sit comfortably for two minutes, without doing anything. If you feel like moving your arm, your leg or your neck, just do it gently. After this waiting time, you can open your eyes. Don't rush this part as the two minutes is allowing you to physiologically come from a very deep state of relaxation to your normal state of wakefulness.

Daylong Stress Relief

Many types of meditation recommend another tool that can be used to reduce stress throughout the day. It is the use of a mantra: a word or phrase that is repeated silently over and over in your mind. Repetition of this word or phrase will quiet your mind, while your body calms down, and you become more focused.

Chapter 7
Nourish Thyself: Foods and Relaxation

Not many years ago, anyone into health foods was automatically labeled a "health nut," an excessive worrier, a hypochondriac. This certainly is changing now as more and more information confirms that the normal U.S. diet, often called a "junk food diet," is the cause of much illness and suffering—and that a health food diet is really better for us. This change has allowed stores like Whole Foods and Trader Joe's to flourish.

However, even with our growing awareness of the importance of eating nourishing foods, the value of a healthy diet still is not stressed as a part of the healthcare system and in medical treatment. In some medical schools, nutrition is covered in only one course. Thus, doctors haven't been trained to look for nutritional answers to illnesses. They attempt to treat patients with prescription medication. The only time nutrition may be consider is when a nutritional deficiency is severe enough to become a disease, as in scurvy, beriberi, pellagra, and the like.

Even though more medical research is validating the role of nutrients in healing, doctors largely ignore the foods, nutrients, and combinations we need for optimum health. Recommended Dietary Allowances (RDAs) developed by Food and Nutrition Board of the National Research Council do not specify what our bodies need for optimum health and wellness.

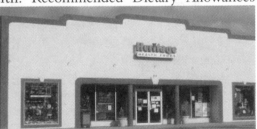

How Accurate Are the RDAs?

In 1974, Senator William Proxmire made a statement in the United States Senate that is still accurate today:

"There are a dozen or more reasons why the so-called RDA is a capricious, unscientific, and illogical standard.

"First and foremost is the unconscionable conflict of interest of those on the Food and Nutrition Board which establishes it. The board is both the creature of the food industry and heavily financed by the food industry. It is in the narrow economic interest of the industry to establish low official RDAs because the lower the RDAs the more nutritional their food products appear.

"The present chairman of the Food and Nutrition Board, for example, occupies an academic chair funded by the Mead Johnson Baby Food Company. He appeared at the FDA vitamin hearings not only as an FDA-Government witness but also on behalf of such firms and groups as Mead Johnson and Abbott Laboratories. He was also scheduled to appear on behalf of the Pet Milk Company and Disillation Products. His research was funded to the tune of about $40,000 by the FDA and he had additional government grants of about $90,000 in the year he appeared for the FDA.

"In the 1974 edition of the Food and Nutrition Board's RDAs, most values that were changed were lowered from previous standards....

"With low RDAs the food companies...can then print tables on their food packages making their products appear to contain a higher level of nutrients than if higher or optimum levels were established.

"A second reason why the RDA standards are suspect is that they have fluctuated capriciously from year to year both in the nutrients listed and in the Recommended Daily Allowance. For example, in the recommendations by the Board for panthothenic acid, a B-complex vitamin, in the period 1964 to 1974, it was not on the 1964 list, was listed at 5 mg. on the next list, was not on the third list, was back at 5 mg. on the fourth list, was doubled to 10 mg. on the fifth list, and was removed completely from the latest 1974 edition.

"In the 1968 RDA list, there were 55 changes in value from the 1964 list, varying from 20 to 700 percent. The latest (1974) list shows similar subjective and unscientific variations.

"Third...there is a very considerable body of scientific evidence that the RDA's are ridiculously low. For example: Folacin. The RDA for folacin for some categories of individuals has varied by 700 percent in the last ten years. The latest pronouncement cut the RDA for children in half. This has come at the very time the Canadian Government's nutritional survey found that half of all Canadians had moderate deficiency levels of folacin in their blood....

"There is strong evidence that the lack of folacin produces congenital deformities and increases the danger of accidental hemorrhage by five-fold."

Senator Proxmire raises some serious doubts about the absolute reliance many persons place on the government's nutritional standards. There will be further discussion of vitamins and minerals later in this chapter.

An infamous study in which mice were found to gain more nutrition from eating cardboard cereal boxes than from the cereals inside points out that we have a lot to learn about the eating habits we take for granted.

Increasing, it is being reported that drug companies are writing reports for researchers about the benefit of certain drugs and suppressing the results of studies with poor results. This, of course, has case doubt on the whole research establishment. There are further questions about experts and consultants who determine the value of various nutrients. It seems many of them are receiving consulting fees from the drug companies that have a financial interest in maintaining the status quo, rather than emphasizing the health value of nutrition.

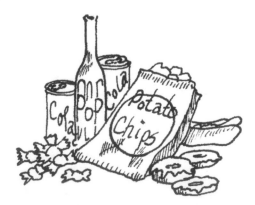

It's Not All in the Mind!

I'll cite two studies that illustrate the profound changes that alterations in diet can bring to a person.

The first was a study of hyperactive children: children who misbehave in class, can't seem to concentrate, have a short attention span, run around nervously, etc. The standard treatment today includes psychoactive drugs, ranging from tranquilizers to amphetamines. No one really knows why these drugs work or fail to work.

When a group of hyperactive children was removed from the typical American diet—and given no drugs--their hyperactivity disappeared. A simple removal of sugar, preservatives, white flour, and chemical additives from their diets transformed them into normal, fun-loving children, able to pay attention and concentrate. When one child on the diet was given a processed cookie by a friend, the ill effects lasted for three days.

The second area involves the use of megavitamin therapy. This is the use of large doses of vitamins to cure certain diseases.

Schizophrenia, a mental illness, was the first area in which megavitamin therapy was employed. In 1952, Abram Hoffer, M.D. and Humphrey Osmond, M.R.C.P. found that nearly 75 percent of their schizophrenic patients improved with vitamin treatment alone. These patients received none of the customary tranquilizers or "anti-psychotic" drugs.

The North Nassau Mental Health Center in Manhasset, Long Island, is a model center for this type of therapy, also known as orthomolecular psychiatry. Some patients enter the center after other treatment methods (drugs, shock treatment, and psychotherapy) have failed for years. Their nutritional needs are analyzed and a regimen prescribed. Most of them leave several weeks later, feeling and acting normally. The center has successfully treated more than 10,000 patients. One of them, a 30-year-old man who suffered from schizophrenia for more than half his life, summed up the experiences of many:

"Megavitamin therapy is a miracle. I'm well. I've been on it more than a year. No more psychotherapy, hospitals, shock treatments, tranquilizers, or drugs. I feel it has corrected an imbalance in me. I'm fine now, and I'm grateful."

Scientists from Oxford University say eating "junk food" has contributed to increased violence over the last fifty years. In a pilot study of 231 prisoners published in 2002 they found violent incidences decreased by more than a third among prisoners who received nutritional supplements. Expanded research will study 1,000 prisoners and the impact of a vitamin-and-mineral supplement, along with fish oil. The study will examine the contribution of omega-3 fatty acids to increasing brain "flexibility," attention spans, and self-control.

For more information about orthomolecular psychiatry, visit www.Schizophrenia.org or contact Huxley Institute for Biosocial Research, 86-B Dorchester Drive, Lakewood, New Jersey 08701.

The Cholesterol Myth

The uproar against cholesterol is a good example of a mass nutrition myth. A substance of vital importance to our bodies, cholesterol is found in particularly high concentrations in the brain and nervous system. The liver of a normal adult manufactures 800 to 1,000 grams of cholesterol each day—70 to 80 percent of the cholesterol circulating in most individuals' bodies. When we don't eat any cholesterol, our livers manufacture more.

Numerous studies done in the past fifty years show that cholesterol-related problems like arteriosclerosis (hardening of the arteries) are caused not by how much cholesterol we take in, but by improper processing of cholesterol in the body. More recent studies have pointed to low-grade infections in the body, which raise homocysteine levels in the body. This ongoing infection may be culprit behind heart disease.

The key to the solution is exercise and other beneficial lifestyle habits, which keep the arteries free of cholesterol deposits and maintain a healthy heart.

The famed Boston Irish Heart Study, for example, examined 500 pairs of Irish brothers, one of whom had immigrated to Boston while the other remained in Ireland. The Ireland-based brothers ate an average of 26 percent more calories per day, including higher levels of cholesterol and saturated fats than their Boston brothers; yet they had lower serum (bloodstream) cholesterol levels and healthier hearts and arteries. What was the Irishmen's secret?

The authors of this study speculated that exercise was a key factor, since most of the Ireland-based brothers did hard physical labor from dawn to dusk, while their Boston brothers held desk jobs. Subsequent studies have confirmed this. The Ireland-based brothers' diets were also notably richer in whole grains.

Cholesterol circulates in the blood in two kinds of packages: low-density lipoproteins (LDLs) and high-density lipoproteins (HDLs). LDLs deliver cholesterol to the tissues—they've been called "the body's oil trucks." Excesses of LDL cholesterol can end up plastered to artery walls. Meanwhile, HDLs carry excess cholesterol away from the tissues to the liver, which will recycle or excrete it. HDLs help to sweep the bloodstream clean of excess cholesterol. Since higher levels of HDL cholesterol protect against heart disease, the goal is to raise the ratio of HDL to LDL cholesterol in the bloodstream.

The single most important factor in doing this seems to be regular exercise, especially aerobic exercise—at least four twenty-minute periods per week. Reducing stress is also significant. And although one need not ban meat and eggs totally from one's diet, well-balanced eating, including lots of whole grains and vegetables and minimizing sweets, white-flour products, and refined foods, is very important. In particular, the following nutrients help to raise HDLs and lower LDLs:

- **Fiber**—specifically the gummy fibers, such as whole oatmeal and oat bran; pectins (found in apples, raw carrots, and other fresh fruits and vegetables); guar gum (found in dried beans); and edible chia seeds.
- **Plant sterols**–Chemical cousins of cholesterol, these fatty alcohols such as beta-sitosterol are found in a wide variety of vegetables, grains, and seeds including soybeans, avocados, barley, cabbage, eggplant, sorghum, sunflower seeds, peanuts, rice, corn, yams, mustard, wheat-germ oil, and vegetable oils.
- **Essential fatty acids**–Omega-3 fatty acids, found in fish and fish oils, soybeans, linseeds and their oils. Lecithin, found in whole grains, legumes, and eggs.
- **Raw garlic or raw-garlic oil**.
- **Yogurt**.

Vitamin C, vitamin E, and the B vitamins are also significant, and recent research shows that proper levels of calcium and magnesium, potassium, and chromium may be important as well.

The Sugar Question

Try this quick food analysis for fun and enlightenment:

List everything you've had to eat or drink in the past 24 hours. Also include things that you usually have but didn't eat during this particular period. List the quantities. Next, estimate how much total sugar was in the foods and beverages you consumed during this period.

Use Table 1 to find out how much sugar you consumed in popular foods. Arrive at a total amount of teaspoons of sugar.

Table 1
So you think you don't eat much sugar?
Here are the approximate amounts of refined sugar (added sugar, in
addition to the sugar naturally present) hidden in popular foods

Food Item	Size/Portion	Approximate Sugar Content in Teaspoons of Granulated Sugar
Beverages		
cola drinks	6 oz bottle or glass	3.5
cordials	3/4 oz glass	1.5
ginger ale	6 oz	5
highball	6 oz glass	2.5
orangeade	8 oz glass	5
root beer	10 oz bottle	4.5
Seven-Up ®	6 oz bottle or glass	3 3/4
soda pop	8 oz bottle	5
sweet cider	1 cup	6
whiskey sour	3 oz glass	1.5
Cakes and Cookies		
angel food	4 oz piece	7
apple sauce cake	4 oz piece	5.5
banana cake	2 oz piece	2
cheese cake	4 oz piece	2
chocolate cake (plain)	4 oz piece	6
chocolate cake (iced)	4 oz piece	10
coffee cake	4 oz piece	4.5
cup cake (iced)	1	6
fruit cake	4 oz piece	5
jelly roll	2 oz piece	2.5
orange cake	4 oz piece	4
pound cake	4 oz piece	5
sponge cake	1 oz piece	2
brownies (unfrosted)	3/4 oz	3
chocolate cookies	1	1.5
Fig Newtons®	1	5
gingersnaps	1	3
macaroons	1	6

nut cookies	1	1.5
oatmeal cookies	1	2
sugar cookies	1	1.5
chocolate éclair	1	7
cream puff	1	2
donut (plain)	1	3
donut (glazed)	1	6

Candies

average milk choc. bar	1 1/2 oz	2.5
chewing gum	1 stick	0.5
chocolate cream	1 piece	2
butterscotch chew	1 piece	1
chocolate mints	1 piece	2
fudge	1 oz square	4.5
gumdrop	1	2
hard candy	4 oz	20
Lifesavers®	1	0.33
peanut brittle	1 oz	3.5

Canned Fruits and Juices

canned apricots	4 halves and 1 T syrup	3.5
canned fruit juices (sweet)	1/2 cup	2
canned peaches	2 halves and 1 T syrup	3.5
fruit salad	1/2 cup	3.5
fruit syrup	2 T	2.5
stewed fruits	1/2 cup	2

Dairy Products

ice cream	1/3 pt (3.5 oz)	3.5
ice cream cone	1	3.5
ice cream soda	1	5
ice cream sundae	1	7
malted milk shake	10 oz glass	5

Jams and Jellies

apple butter	1T	1
jelly	1T	4.6
orange marmalade	1T	4.6
peach butter	1T	1
strawberry jam	1T	4

Desserts, Miscellaneous

apple cobbler	1/2 cup	3
blueberry cobbler	1/2 cup	3
custard	1/2 cup	2
French pastry	4 oz piece	5
fruit gelatin	1/2 cup	4.5
apple pie	1 slice (average)	7
apricot pie	1 slice (average)	7
berry pie	1 slice (average)	10
butterscotch pie	1 slice (average)	4
cherry pie	1 slice (average)	10
cream pie	1 slice (average)	4
lemon pie	1 slice (average)	7
mince meat pie	1 slice (average)	4
peach pie	1 slice (average)	7
prune pie	1 slice (average)	6
pumpkin pie	1 slice (average)	5
rhubarb pie	1 slice (average)	4
banana pudding	1/2 cup	2
bread pudding	1/2 cup	1.5
chocolate pudding	1/2 cup	4
cornstarch pudding	1/2 cup	2.5
date pudding	1/2 cup	7
fig pudding	1/2 cup	7
Grape Nuts® pudding	1/2 cup	2
plum pudding	1/2 cup	4
rice pudding	1/2 cup	5
tapioca pudding	1/2 cup	3
berry tart	1 cup	10
blancmange	1/2 cup	5
brown Betty	1/2 cup	3
plain pastry	4 oz piece	3
sherbet	1/2 cup	9

Syrups, Sugars, and Icings

brown sugar	1 T	3★
chocolate icing	1 oz	5
chocolate sauce	1 T	3.5
corn syrup	1 T	3★
granulated sugar	1 T	3★
honey	1 T	3★
Karo® syrup	1 T	3★
maple syrup	1 T	5★
molasses	1 T	3.5★
white icing	1 oz	5★

★ actual sugar content

Surprised? So you didn't know that a 12-ounce Coke has seven teaspoons of sugar in it? Did you ever imagine that the jelly on your morning toast had four to six teaspoons of sugar or that the chocolate cake with icing had ten teaspoons? Would you drink a cup of plain sugar? Of course not! Yet, we consume a tremendous amount of this substance without knowing it.

Since 1909, sugar consumption has increased 70 percent. The average American diet now contains about 150 pounds of sugar per year, up 25 pounds since 1970. This means that 15 to 25 percent of the total calories consumed a day are from sugar, but sugar provides no nutrition at all. Though it can be burned as energy, we don't need it. We get plenty of fuel from other foods. In fact, the human body was not designed to process refined sugars. Most sugar we eat gets stored as fat. Most important, we can only have a certain number of calories per day. When we eat empty sugar, with no vitamins, no minerals, no fiber, no protein, and no fat, we're passing up some other, nourishing food that we probably need for our health. With increasing levels of obesity and type 2 diabetics in this country, our intake of sugar is just worsening the situation.

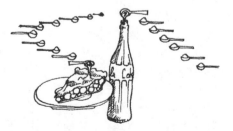

Some authorities feel that sugar is not actually a food, but a chemical, since it has to undergo tremendous processing to arrive in its white, pure, granulated form. Harvard nutritionist Jean Mayer has stated that sugar, which was once an additive, is now being viewed in our society as a "new food"—but it's a food our bodies cannot tolerate.

Some people have switched to brown sugar, thinking that would reduce their sugar consumption. Actually, brown sugar is white sugar, colored and flavored with six to eight percent molasses. All other sugars like turbinado, raw sugar, and the like are almost identical to refined white sugar! Any color or flavor was added after refinement into white sugar...because it's against the law to sell unprocessed sugar in the United States.

Sugar seems to trigger or contribute to many illnesses. It has been linked to coronary heart disease, mental illness, dental caries, diabetes, hypoglycemia, obesity, and others.

So what should you substitute for sugar? Artificial sweeteners are risky because their long-term chemical effects on the body are unknown. Sweeteners that can be used are honey, blackstrap molasses, sorghum, and unsweetened fruit juice. All of these substances contain nutrients within them: in other words, they are still alive. These nutrients aid the body in its functioning.

Table 2 shows comparative nutritional values of sugar, honey and molasses, as determined by the U.S. Department of Agriculture.

Table 2
Sugars, Honey, and Molasses Compared

	White Sugar	Brown Sugar	Molasses, Blackstrap	Honey strained	Maple Sugar
Minerals - mg.					
Calcium	0	85	684	5	143
Phosphorus	0	19	84	6	11
Iron	0.1	3.4	16.1	0.5	1.4
Potassium	3	344	2927	51	242
Sodium	1	30	96	5	14
Vitamins					
Thiamin	0	0.01	0.11	trace	–
Riboflavin	0	0.03	0.19	0.04	–
Niacin	0	0.2	2	0.3	–

Source: "Composition of Foods," Agriculture Handbook No. 8, USDA

Fortunately, there are other alternatives to sugar available today. One is Agave nectar, which is similar in taste and texture to honey. It is 1.4 times sweeter than sugar, but has nearly half the amount of carbohydrates.

Another option is Stevia, available in health food stores and in the natural foods aisles of many supermarkets. Stevia is from South America and has been used for thousands of years as a sweetener. It's around 150 to 250 times sweeter than sugar. Because of that you'll have to experiment with the amount you'll need. And the best part is it has no calories.

Xylitol offers the same sweetness as sugar but with 40 percent fewer calories and none of the negative tooth decay or insulin release effects of sugar.

Lo Han is made from a fruit from China. It has no measurable caloric value and a very low glycemic index. It does not cause sweet or food cravings, nor does it stimulate fat storage. Finally, Lo Han does not raise blood sugar and is safe for most diabetics and hypoglycemics.

Foods and Stress Relief

Do you eat when you're under stress? Go ahead—admit it. You're certainly not alone. Experts say that most people overeat when under stress because we've learned that food brings (short-term) comfort. Stress can also deplete the body's energy reserves, so we reach for sugar and high-fat foods.

Fresh fruits and veggies; supplemental vitamins like B complex, C, and E; and even dark chocolate, which contains magnesium, can be helpful in relieving stress. You might be aware that drinking a glass of warm milk before bedtime will quiet the mind and prepare you for sleep. But did you know that a handful of pistachio nuts can ease your stress? This may sound nutty, but it's true. Nutritionists at Penn State University had students eat pistachio nuts daily for a month. They found this kept the students' blood pressure down in stressful situations. When they upped the amount to two handfuls every day, the students' arteries relaxed, which may lighten how hard the heart has to pump.

Hypoglycemia: Everyone's Problem?

The foods you eat each day have a significant impact on how you feel that day—relaxed or tense, energetic or weary, calm or anxious, pleasant or irritable. You may be tired, depressed, or even in pain because the foods you eat are playing havoc with your blood sugar level.

The body needs to maintain a particular level of sugar in the blood, just as it needs to maintain a particular oxygen level. Depending on your body chemistry, you need between 50 and 150 mg. of glucose (the body's sugar) per 100 cc. of blood at all times—less than two teaspoonfuls in the entire body! The proper blood sugar level is crucial, especially for brain functioning; we literally cannot "think straight" if it's too high or too low.

Sweets and processed carbohydrates can have a devastating effect on blood sugar and consequently on one's physical energy and emotional state. By processed carbohydrates, I mean candy, soft drinks, sugared drinks, and refined flour products such as cakes, cookies, breads, cereals, crackers, and pasta. Even whole-grain products, honey, or molasses (all healthy in other ways) can upset your blood sugar if eaten in large quantities.

When sweets or processed carbohydrates hit the stomach—anyone's stomach—they are instantly converted to glucose, which hits the blood stream in minutes. You can feel it—that much-touted "burst of energy" after eating a sweet. You may feel revved up, nervous, excited. But the body needs a stable—not seesaw—level of blood sugar to function. Actually, your brain is saying, "Oh, no…what hit me?!" Your pancreas is registering, "Emergency!…Sugar overload!…Emergency!"

As more and more glucose comes out of your stomach into your blood during the next few minutes, your pancreas pours out insulin to process it, keeping your system out of the danger of having too much sugar in your system at the same time. However, the pancreas has no way of knowing when the sugar flood will end. This means that the pancreas will overreact, producing too much insulin, which in turn removes too much sugar from the system. In some people this reaction is mild; in some it's drastic. Either way, the outcome is low blood sugar. Low? That's right. You are left, an hour after eating a sweet, with low blood sugar and a ravenous appetite. If you're like most people, you try to satisfy that appetite with another sweet—and the cycle starts again. Your blood sugar level becomes like a yo-yo going up and down all day long—sugar in your breakfast cereal, a donut for mid-morning snack, a soft drink with lunch, a candy bar for your afternoon snack, and dessert after dinner.

The well-documented results of low blood sugar range from fatigue, nervousness, anxiety, depression, lack of motivation, irrationality, colds, muscle pains, asthma, and hay fever, all the way up to heart palpitations, coma, and mental illness—complete with hallucinations. The more severe and chronic the addition to sugar, the more side effects you'll have.

Most of these symptoms are the familiar complaints for which we can never seem to find a cause or cure. Some doctors estimate that hypoglycemia affects 50 to 80 percent of Americans mildly to moderately and often is not diagnosed. As for more severe cases, E.M. Abrahamson, M.D., and A.W. Pezet, two authoritative writers on the subject, said, "Persons who at last were found to be suffering from hypoglycemia have been treated for coronary thrombosis and other heart ailments, brain tumor, epilepsy, gall bladder disease, appendicitis, hysteria, and every sort of neurosis. They have been told repeatedly that their trouble is 'all in the mind' and sent to the psychoanalyst."

How does one acquire low blood sugar? According to these authors, one can create this illness simply by eating the modern North American diet, with its sweets and carbohydrates. Ingesting lots of sweets teaches our pancreas to respond to any upswing in blood sugar as a drastic emergency. The only way to desensitize and normalize our insulin production and our blood sugar is to change our eating habits. For children, it makes sense not to let them become sugar addicts in the first place. (Expectant mothers delivering their babies in hospitals should instruct the hospitals not to give sugar-water to their newborn children.)

In case you don't think any of this applies to you...do you drink coffee? Caffeine has the same effect as sugar. It stimulates the adrenal glands to produce adrenaline, the "fight-or-flight" hormone, and adrenaline in turn triggers the liver to pour stored sugar (glycogen) into the bloodstream. The pancreas reacts, and the seesaw starts again. That's why so many people go through their workdays fighting off fatigue, feeling half-asleep. They munch sweets and gulp coffee by the hour in the mistaken notion that this increases their energy. Actually, these substances sap energy by decreasing the blood sugar. By the end of the day, these workers are worn out. They think: "Why am I always so tired? This job is exhausting me."

If you've experienced any of the complaints that could be related to hypoglycemia, or if you're simply interested in trying out a high-energy, fatigue-reducing diet, follow these guidelines for two to four weeks. It can't hurt...and might do wonders for you!

1. No sugared drinks, candy, commercial cereals, ice cream, cake, cookies, pasta, potato chips, or crackers. (If you think you can't live without sweets and breadstuffs, remember that the craving for these substances may well be caused by the low blood sugar that results from eating them in the first place. For many people, the craving disappears when they're on this diet.)

2. Eat little or no white bread, potatoes, fruit juices, and processed grains. If you must have some, eat in small quantities at a meal with proteins and vegetables. You can have moderate amounts of whole grains, beans, and whole fruits. Use only whole-grain breads. If you must have cereal, try whole rolled oats or unprocessed bran sweetened with raisins or fresh fruit.

3. When you want something sweet, eat a piece of fresh fruit. Fruit is high in carbohydrate, but its absorption into the system is slowed by its fiber content, and its concentration is diluted by its high water content.

4. Eat relatively small meals, even if that means increasing your (healthy) snacks. Snack on fruits, nuts, sunflower seeds, vegetables, unsweetened nut butters, cheeses, etc.

5. Avoid caffeine—coffee, cola drinks and teas—as much as possible. (Decaffeinated coffee and herb teas are okay.)

6. Initially avoid all alcohol. After two weeks without alcohol, you can begin to drink red wine, limiting your amount to no more than two glasses per day. While red wine has been found to contain nutrients that aid in our living longer, take care to limit your consumption as alcohol is digested as a pure sugar.

After two to four weeks of this diet, mildly hypoglycemic persons can add back modest amounts of juices and natural sweeteners and can increase their intake of whole-grain carbohydrates. By then, you should be developing an awareness of your body and your moods, which will help you regulate yourself.

Natural sweeteners are honey, molasses, maple syrup, sorghum, dates, figs, dried (but not glazed!) fruits, and unsweetened fruit and vegetable juices. Whole-grain carbohydrates include anything made strictly with whole-grain flour, including cookies, cakes, bread, and pasta.

Remember that it's best not to eat a lot of these kinds of foods at one time, and to eat them with other types of foods. Proteins, fats, and the fiber in whole grains and vegetables help to slow down the stomach's digestion of carbohydrates so that the sugar has less of an impact on the body. As a matter of fact, if you are going to have a sweet, have it with a meal. However, you still want to limit the amount, as most desserts and sweets have minimal nutritional value. The same advice applies to caffeine and alcohol—use in moderation and accompanied by other foods.

White Flour vs. Whole-Wheat Flour

A long time ago it was discovered by millers that by taking the wheat germ out of the wheat, they would get a product that would not turn rancid. It was of little concern to them that they were also removing all the nutritional value and fiber content of the flour. This "de-natured" white flour will not support even bacteria life—that's why it won't spoil!

It's a little know fact that during the two world wars, several countries, including Denmark and Norway, stopped milling white flour, so that only whole-wheat flour was available. These nations also reduced or banned meat consumption. Research has shown a tremendous correlation between the drop in heart disease during this period—until white flour and meats were reinstated.

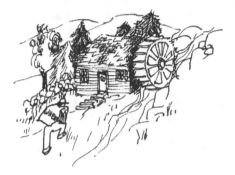

In the milling process, vitamins and minerals are removed from the flour. To make so-called "enriched" flour, the miller adds four or five artificial vitamins and minerals to white flour. Mathematically, we have suffered a major loss of nutrients (See Table 3). In addition, all of the fiber has been removed and the protein value of the flour has been reduced.

In choosing whole-wheat bread, be sure to read the label. Products labeled "made with whole wheat" are often refined. Check for the percentage of whole grains in the product. Make sure whole grains are listed among the first items in the products ingredient list.

Table 3
Whole-Wheat Flour Compared to White Flour

100 g. or 3.5 oz of Flour	Whole Wheat Flour	White Flour	% of the amount supplied by Whole Wheat Flour	Enriched White Flour	% of the amount supplied by Whole Wheat Flour
Protein	13.3 g.	10.5 g.	79%	10.5 g.	79%
Minerals					
Calcium	41 mg	16 mg	39%	16 mg	39%
Phosphorous	372 mg	87 mg	23%	87 mg	39%
Iron	3.3 mg	0.8 mg	24%	2.9 mg	88%
Potassium	370 mg	95 mg	26%	95 mg	26%
Sodium	3 mg	2 mg	67%	2 mg	67%
Vitamins					
Thiamin	0.55 mg	0.06 mg	11%	0.44 mg	80%
Riboflavin	0.12 mg	0.05 mg	42%	0.26 mg	216%
Niacin	4.3 mg	0.9 mg	21%	3.5 mg	81%

Source: "Composition of Foods," Agriculture Handbook, No.8, USDA

Fiber In Your Diet

Fiber gives the digestive system necessary exercise and keeps the foods you've consumed moving along, thus alleviating constipation. Some researchers have found that cancer of the colon may result from sluggish bowel action, due to cancer-causing wastes remaining in contact with the colon walls for too long a period of time. Adequate fiber in the diet has been credited with reduced incidences of gall bladder disease, hemorrhoids, and varicose veins.

The original study on fiber was done by Dr. Neil S. Painter, a London surgeon. He studied the effects of bran fiber on patients with diverticular disease. In this painful, common ailment, pockets or sacs are formed in the colon as a result of too much pressure (constipation, hard stools, etc.). When these patients used bran fiber, they had soft stools and easy defecation without straining. Constipation disappeared. The use of laxatives decreased dramatically. While bran fiber can sometimes cause stomach gas, this symptom will generally disappeared within three weeks.

There are two types of fiber: soluble and insoluble. Soluble fiber assists the liver by binding with bile acids, helping to lower total cholesterol, including LDL cholesterol. It also prolongs the time it takes for the stomach to empty, slowing the release and absorption of sugar. Insoluble fiber moves bulk through the intestines to remove toxic waste more quickly and prevent constipation. It also controls and balances the pH in the intestines.

While you can get some fiber from fruits, vegetables, and whole grains, you have many choices for adding additional fiber to your diet. Twenty grams of bran have the same bulking effect as 200 to 300 grams of most other foodstuffs. In addition, you can purchase cereals with significant amounts of fiber, orange juice that retains the pulp.

How much bran do you need? Just adding two to three tablespoons of raw bran to your diet each day is all that is necessary. Start with one tablespoon per day (some at each meal or all at once), and gradually increase the amount to two to three tablespoons per day. You can add the bran to cereal, yogurt, soup, casseroles, ground meat, bread, muffins, pancakes, etc. Always have some liquid with the bran. Another way to get your fiber is to consume bran tablets purchased from a health food store.

Bran is also great for dieting. Take raw bran with a glass of water shortly before each meal. The bran expands to partially fill the stomach so that you don't want as much food. In addition, British physicians such as Dr. K. W. Heaton of the University Department of Medicine in Bristol have found that fiber can slow down calorie absorption, allowing the body to excrete an extra 200 or more calories each day.

Ground flax seeds and chia seeds are also healthy sources of fiber. Chia seeds (the kind that you can eat, not grow) are worth considering because they have 38% more fiber and 247% more calcium (that number is not an error) than flax seeds. They are also rich in omega-3 fatty acids.

Additives:
What You Don't Know Could Hurt You

Why is diet cola bad for you? Why should you avoid something labeled "artificial" or "imitation?"

Chemical additives are not natural substances; they are synthetic. There are two problems with additives: most of them are untested, and many may be carcinogenic.

Many additives have not been tested for their safety. Few have been tested for long-term effects: what they do to a person over ten, twenty, or fifty years of consumption. In addition, when each substance is tested, it is tested in isolation. This testing ignores the synergistic process—the fact

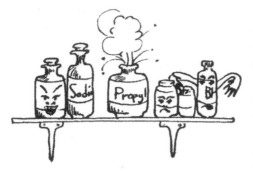 that chemicals in combination can have a totally different effect than one chemical alone. How do these additives react with each other in our bodies? How do they react with other chemicals we take in through our lungs, in our water, in medications? We have no idea. One or two of these substances probably would not be a problem; the problem is the enormous number of these unknowns, and their increasing usage by the food industry to bolster color, flavor, and freshness after natural color and flavor have been reduced by commercial growing and processing methods. Another concern is what genetically modified foods may be doing to our bodies and our environment.

The point of this discussion is not to criticize all technology and invention. But we have seen that seemingly helpful or supposedly innocuous substances (certain chemicals, plastics, detergents, insecticides, industrial wastes) can wreak havoc on our water supply, our air, our food supply, animal life, and our bodies. The damages, when they have appeared, have been devastating–a dead lake, a polluted water supply, the high mercury content of many fish, the high chemical content in the milk of nursing mothers. It is time to begin using technology with foresight, especially as it relates to our own health. Until this foresight becomes standard commercial procedure, we can protect ourselves by demanding and purchasing foods without chemical additives.

The additive problem was famously illustrated in the 1970s by the case of Red Dye No. 2. There was a twenty-year controversy about whether or not this chemical could cause cancer. During this time, it was continuously added to foods and alcoholic beverages. Finally, the U.S. Food and Drug Administration, which today still moves at glacial speeds, had it removed from the market as a potential cancer-causing agent. Red Dye No. 2 is just one of many additives tested and deemed unsafe after they had been added to our foods for some time.

Consider the more recent issue of trans fats. Used commonly before 2006 to enhance the flavor, texture, and shelf life of many processed foods, most scientists now agree that eating trans fats raises the risk of heart disease and type 2 diabetes. New York City became the first city to ban all trans fats from foods sold in New York.

A word of caution on trans fats and the role of the FDA: Even if the label on the product claims that it has 0 percent trans fats, this might not be true. The FDA allows a manufacturer to claim that the product has no trans fats, while it allows up to ½ gram of trans fats to be in every serving. What does this mean? Well, assume you are eating potato chips, and the label says a serving is ten chips. You eat 40 chips. This means it is possible that you just unknowingly consumed two grams of trans fats. So much for the FDA protecting the consumer. I'll discuss trans fats more in the information below.

Here are some common food additives in processed foods to which you may want to pay particular attention.

- **Artificial colorings** have been suspected of causing increased hyperactivity in children. Yellow Die No. 5 may worsen asthma symptoms.
- **High fructose corn syrup** is sweeter and cheaper than cane sugar. Some experts are concerned that the body metabolizes high fructose corn syrup in such a way as to raise the risk of obesity and type 2 diabetes more than sugar. High fructose corn syrup is being used as a key ingredient in more and more foods and beverages. Keep in mind that neither sugar nor high fructose corn syrup offers nutritional benefits to the body and should be limited.
- **Trans fats** are created by adding hydrogen to vegetable oil. They raise the level of LDL "bad" cholesterol, increasing the risk of heart disease. Unlike saturated fats, they also lower HDL "good" cholesterol and may do more damage, says the American Heart Association. How can you tell if a product that is labeled 0 grams trans fat actually contains it? Look on the ingredients list for the words "partially hydrogenated." Any oil that is partially hydrogenated is a trans fat. Also, limit your overall daily fat intake. Many fried foods and baked goods are prepared with a significant amount of trans fats.
- **Aspartame** is an artificial sweetener that has raised various health concerns, including causing cancer, seizures, headaches, mood disturbances, and reduced mental performance. Aspartame is also suspected of contributing to concerns such as fibromyalgia, spasms, shooting pains, numbness in the leg, cramps, vertigo, dizziness, headaches, tinnitus, joint pain, depression, anxiety attacks, slurred speech, blurred vision, and memory loss.

- **Monosodium glutamate**, or MSG, can be found in thousands of processed foods from soup to crackers to meats. It's even in infant formulas and baby foods. MSG can be disguised on ingredients labels as broth, casein, hydrolyzed vegetable protein, autolyzed gelatin, yeast extract, malted barley, rice syrup and brown rice syrup. In his book Excitotoxins: The Taste That Kills, Dr. Russell Blaylock says MSG may give us more than just headaches. It may actually be poisoning us. Dr. Blaylock explains that MSG is an excitotoxin, which means it overexcites your cells to the point of damaging them. This makes it act as a poison. In addition, since the 1960s, scientists have known that MSG causes obesity.
- **Sodium benzoate**, added as a preservative to foods and drinks, may increase hyperactivity in children. When used in soft drinks, it may react with added vitamin C to become benzene, a cancer-causing agent.
- **Sodium nitrite**, used in curing meat, is suspected of contributing to gastric cancer.

Why Eat Organic?

Non-organic, conventionally grown crops are developed and bred for a variety of factors—color, size, and rapid growth (so that another crop may be grown in the same season). These crops are not developed with high-quality nutrition in mind, and the other factors involved may actually conflict with their ability to offer good nutrition.

Additionally, in this country, we also have to deal with genetically modified foods (or GMOs, for genetically modified organisms), which scientists are putting into farm production without a clear picture of the dangers to the environment and to our bodies that they may present. The government under President G.W. Bush decided that foods labels don't have state that they contain GMO foods, preventing consumers from voting with their dollars for eating these foods—or not! The European Union has a much better approach. They have banned GMO foods from being sold in the EU.

Conventionally grown crops are grown on land used constantly to maximum capacity. This means the soil that the crop has been grown on may have been depleted of its natural minerals. There may be no iron, calcium, zinc, magnesium, or any of a dozen other trace elements necessary for optimum functioning of the human body. The standard fertilizers used to grow these crops add only nitrogen, potassium, and phosphorus to the soil.

Second, non-organic crops have been sprayed with powerful pesticides and insecticides. As with food additives, we don't know which ones will eventually prove unsafe: remember DDT? Non-organic farmers also use powerful weed-killers, which are generally designed to kill any plant life other than a specific group of vegetables. What might these chemicals do to our bodies?

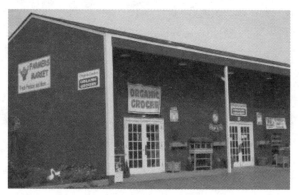

Organic farmers depend on good crop rotation to improve soil quality, increase yields, and manage pests. They also try to rebalance the soil with the proper minerals. Only natural methods of pest control are employed on crops, such as using plant extracts, and growing certain crops and flowers side by side as a way to protect each other. Some of these methods have been known for thousands of years. In addition, maintaining the soil in a healthy state seems to give plants natural protection against insect pests.

Fortunately, many stores, from your local supermarket to large chains, are carrying a wide variety of organic meat and produce now, making it much easier to eat safe and healthy food. While organic foods may appear to cost more at the cash register, they have many more nutrients in them compared to conventional foods. You would need to buy many times the amount of conventionally grown food to get the nutritional benefits found in organic foods. You will also avoid health concerns since there were no pesticides or insecticides used on the organic foods. Additionally, organic vegetables actually stay fresh a lot longer than non-organic ones.

In these difficult times, more Americans are growing their own vegetables (keep in mind the organic White House garden that Michelle Obama started) and shopping at farmers markets. Keep in mind that many small growers at farmers markets cannot afford to have a government agency certify their crops "organic." Talk to them. They may assure you that they use sustainable growing practices that are just as good as organic. If they are local, then their foods are probably better for the environment than even those grown by the huge organic farming industry and trucked thousands of miles to your market.

A word about the terms "natural" versus "organic." Research is showing that American consumers are coming to trust a label that says a food is "natural" more than one that says "organic." There is no legal definition of a "natural" food. The food industry use of the term "natural" may indicate that a food has been minimally processed and is free of preservatives. The label "organic" on a product means it has met a strict definition of how it was grown or raised.

Vitamins

While there are more and more studies in the mainstream medical journals recognizing that vitamins and minerals play a crucial role in health, many doctors are still quite skeptical and/or uninformed when it comes to considering the use of supplements for individual patients.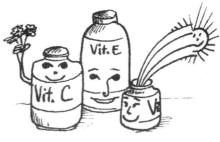

Let me relate my own experience: I have always had extremely cold hands and feet. When I became a vegetarian (no, you don't have to become a vegetarian) the problem became even worse. During the winter, I'd be indoors writing, and my hand would cramp up from being so cold. This situation finally forced me to experiment with vitamins. The result of this is that my extremities are warm 80 percent of the time, even during the middle of the winter.

While seeing a doctor for a regular check-up, I asked the doctor if there were any vitamins that I could take to be 100 percent warm, In response, I got a lecture on the total uselessness of vitamins to correct circulation problems. The doctor's advice? Learn to live with the problem. (I did not mention that vitamins had already corrected most of it.)

Another true story illustrates how effective vitamins can be. Recently, I drove to a conference with Debbie, a colleague in the travel business. During the drive, Debbie told me that she had been experiencing severe depressions at least once a day. The depressions appeared to be unrelated to things happening in her life, She could have a day full of good experiences and still become depressed. As could be expected, this was causing her a great deal of concern.

I questioned her about her diet It turned out to be a "typical" North American diet of processed foods, sweet snacks, white sugar and flour, chemicals, and preservatives. I told her that her problem might be a vitamin deficiency. Since she was open to trying some remedy, I gave her a supply of my vitamins to last the three days of the conference, (See next page for recommended amounts.)

On the third day of the conference, she told me that she felt great and that she felt like a new person. She had not been depressed even once during the entire conference, despite the fact that there were many problems she had to deal with at the conference. Debbie told me that she had even tried to get depressed just to see if she could do it—and she could not! When she returned home, friends remarked that she was totally different. Her co-workers even called to thank me for the change in Debbie. I told them the vitamins were responsible, not me. Debbie's boss was so impressed that she now keeps vitamins next to the water cooler.

The normal ways in which foods are grown, processed, preserved, stored, shipped, and cooked result in vast losses of vitamins and minerals. As much as 40 to 50 percent of the B and C vitamins in foods is lost this way. Thus, it is difficult to get the necessary amounts of vitamins and minerals for optimum health from the things we eat.

In June of 2002, a landmark study analyzing 36 years of data in the Journal of the American Medical Association concluded that everyone needs a daily multivitamin regardless of age or health.

While there is still controversy about whether supplements are absorbed by the body in the same way as nutrients from food, a wide range of studies find that supplements can play a role in positively altering health and well-being.

The following suggestions for vitamins and minerals to consume daily come from Dr. Michael Colgan, an Australian-born physician who now heads his own institute, the Colgan Institute of Nutritional Science in San Diego, California, specializing in research in sports medicine. His groundbreaking research shows how different vitamins and minerals work together in the body, how supplements can be used to treat various ailments, and how to determine your individual supplement needs based on diet, lifestyle, and health factors.

The amounts listed here represent Dr. Colgan's "basic formula." The lower amounts are for someone weighing 120 pounds or less; the higher numbers are for someone weighing 180 pounds. If you weigh more than 180 pounds, double the lower figures. To further refine these amounts to your needs, see Dr. Colgan's book The New Nutrition: Medicine for the Millennium. Where his amounts differ greatly from other research I consider to be credible, I have listed the alternative amounts in brackets.

Daily Suggested Supplements
- B-complex tablets, or combination of tablets, that add up to:
  - 10-15 milligrams (mg.) each of B1 and B2
  - 50-75 mg. B3 (niacin or niacinamide)
  - 20-30 mg. each B5 (panthothenic acid) and B6
  - 20-30 micrograms (mcg.) B12
  - 100-150 mg. each choline and inositol [Alternative: up to 1000 mg. each]
  - 200-300 mcg. folic acid
  - 500-750 mcg. biotin [Alt.: 25 mcg.].
  - 50-75 mg. PABA.
- Vitamin C: 1,000-1,500 mg., with 100-150 mg. bioflavonoids.
- Beta Carotine 20 -30 mg.,
- Vitamin D3 1000-5000 units
- Vitamin E: 200-300 units [Alt.: up to 800 units].
- Minerals:
  - 1000-1500 mg. calcium with 1/ 2 as much magnesium as calcium, and 2/5 (40 percent) as much phosphorus as calcium
  - 10-15 mg. iron
  - 1-1.5 mg. copper
  - 5-7.5 mg. each zinc and manganese [Alt.: 15-30 mg. zinc]
  - 25-37 mcg. each selenium and chromium [Alt.: 200 mcg. Selenium]
  - 50-75 mcg. each iodine and molybdenum [Alt.: 15 mcg. iodine].

Divide your daily amount of vitamin and mineral pills into two or three portions, as they will absorb better when taken over the course of several meals. Always take supplements just after a good-sized meal, with a large glass of cool liquid. (Vitamins and minerals work with food in the body. Hot beverages can destroy some of their potency.)

While this might seem like a large quantity to take each day, many of these amounts are available in standard combinations. Check health-food stores, food cooperatives, and mail-order advertisements in magazines like Prevention for the combinations, prices, and quality you prefer.

Keep in mind that each person is biochemically unique as to their exact vitamin and mineral needs; it may be necessary to adjust recommended amounts to suit you. Tune in to your body to see what feels best. (See "Body Talk" section, p, 103.).

Several good options of where to purchase your vitamins and minerals include:

- The Whitaker Wellness Institute: www.DrWhitaker.com
- Village Green Apothecary: www.MyVillageGreen.com. Their pharmacists can consult with you about your specific needs. They specialize in custom compounding of vitamins, minerals, and prescription drugs from a nutritionist or physician's orders.
- The Heritage Store: www.HeritageStore.com
- Dr Joseph Mercola: www.Mercola.com

A nutritionist or nutritionally oriented physician can help determine your exact vitamin and mineral requirements. S/he may prescribe a hair, blood, or tissue analysis, a glucose tolerance test, and other measures to plan the best diet for you. To find holistic or nutritionally aware doctors in your area, visit the American Holistic Medical Association at www. HolisticMedicine.org.

A Word about Shopping

Always read the labels and be aware of the ingredients in the products you buy—no matter where you buy them, no matter what the larger words on the package say. As I discussed, not everything marked "All Natural" is really healthy. I've picked up loaves of "natural" bread that contained sugar and "wheat flour" bread that listed enriched (white) flour as the major ingredient.

Not everything in a health food store (even Whole Foods) is sugarless, whole grain, organic, or healthy. If you are trying to avoid sweet snacks to even out your blood sugar, an all-natural honey-granola bar is not necessarily a good thing to eat. You'll need to read the label to make your determination.

Chapter 8
Herbs to Soothe and Relax

Herbs have been used for centuries as natural relaxants and medicines. The herbs that act specifically on the nervous system to relax and calm the body are called "nervines." The herbs mentioned herein can be bought at certain pharmacies and most health food stores without a prescription. Since these herbs are usually taken 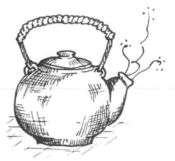 internally as teas and pills, it is important to recognize the potency and purpose of each tea or pill and use them with care.

Nature has provided these substances that may help heal many different ailments. Some herbs can be used anytime and in a general way to help one to relax. But some work in a more specific way to affect a cure, such as by speeding up the action of the digestive tract or detoxifying the liver to restore the body to a more balanced state.

My all-time favorite is chamomile tea. Chamomile is a great relaxer and, if used before bedtime or before a massage, it helps one to sink easily into the deeper levels of relaxation. It also does a great job of calming an upset stomach. If you are using loose teas, you steep the flowers in boiled (not boiling) water for three to five minutes and then serve either plain or with honey. It's important to use only a teaspoon of tea per cup, at most. Don't steep too long or the tea will be too strong and taste bitter. Strain all the teas except chamomile; it's fun to have a few of the flowers bobbing in the teacup. If you're using a tea bag, dunk the bag about thirty times to release more of the tea's potency.

Chamomile can also be used externally in a massage oil: heat up some almond oil mixed with some favorite massage oil and a few chamomile flowers. Pour this into a bowl and begin your massage. The fragrance of the Chamomile flowers makes it aromatic.

Mint teas give a very peaceful and quieting "high" feeling. They are also very aromatic, and I haven't found anyone yet who didn't enjoy them. They relieve "gas" pains in the stomach, soothe the nerves, and can calm someone in an agitated state. My favorite mint tea is spearmint. It can be used alone or combined with chamomile. Licorice root, a very sweet herb that can be used in combination with many others, goes particularly well with mint. Use sparingly.

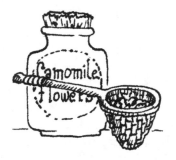

Another very useful tea is sage. It relieves pain, increases circulation, and quiets the nerves. Do not steep this tea too long.

Blue cohosh helps to relieve menstrual cramps.

Still another tea to use by itself is lobelia. Lobelia should be used conservatively. While it can be a stimulant and a muscle relaxant, it is also an intense depressant if used too often or in too high a dosage. Drink only one cup a day.

In cases of anxiety or insomnia, hops is probably the most potent cure. Hops is a main ingredient in beer and has been known for centuries to have great natural tranquilizing properties. Pillows have been stuffed with it to help induce sleep. I like to use hops combined with scullcap and catnip (other potent nervines) to produce a calm "floating" level of consciousness. This combination can put the most worried person to sleep.

Other herbs you can use are blue violet and red clover. There is what I call the "rainbow cure" for cases of general nervousness. You will combine red clover, blue violet, and goldenseal in the ratio 3-3-1. These three herbs combine wonderfully, but please use honey. Goldenseal (a powerful antibiotic that proves useful in many illnesses) tastes very bitter and medicine-y otherwise. This tea will also purify the blood and strengthen the internal organs.

As you can see, certain herbs can be combined. These are called "synergistic" herbs. These herbs blend into each other and create new flavors, powers, and cures that could not be obtained from any one by itself. Here are some of my favorite synergistic herb combinations:

Lemongrass and mint cool the body in summer and ease tension as they refresh. Sassafras, wintergreen, and mugwort make a great muscle relaxant. In hysterical states use valerian, hops, and scullcap. In the case of high blood pressure use snakeroot, black cohosh, and pennyroyal. For headache, use rosemary and yarrow.

Many people may suffer anxiety, tension, and restless leg syndrome because of a lack of calcium in their diets. This also happens when the elements that aid in assimilating calcium in the body are lacking. Herbs such as chamomile, comfrey, and okra contain calcium; and comfrey is said to aid in the use of it in the body.

Two varieties of ginseng, Panax and Siberian, can have a beneficial impact on stress. Studies over more than forty years have validated the ability of Panax ginseng to increase energy level, mood, sexuality, sleep, and work performance. Siberian ginseng has been shown to help reduce chronic fatigue syndrome, decrease fatigue levels, and repair the body's immune functions. The recommended dosage for Panax is 75 to 150 mg per day, and for Siberian it is 150 to 300 mg per day. The only warning for side effects is for Panax ginseng, which in high doses, can cause insomnia, high blood pressure, and heart palpitations.

One herb that gets used differently is mugwort. Stuff mugwort into your pillow and sleep on it for vivid, colorful, memorable dreams. For a truly euphoric evening, sleep on a mugwort and hops pillow, after you've had a Shiatsu massage with chamomile oil rubbed on your body, after drinking a cup of hot sage tea, after a warm bath! Ahhhhhhh...

Yogi Tea

Yogi tea is the name for an unusually relaxing and delightful tea. As you'll see from the recipe, most of the ingredients can be found on your own spice rack. If you drink several cups of the tea, you will discover why I call it an unusual tea. Experiment with it, you will like it! You can now buy a brand called Yogi Tea, which also has unique mixtures of teas in them.

While the following recipe is for one cup of the tea, I would suggest preparing a large batch. Whatever you do not use can be refrigerated until the milk is added.

To make one cup of Yogi tea, place the following ingredients in a pot with a tight-fitting lid:
8 whole cloves
8 cardamom seeds (crushed)
6 black pepper corns (whole)
1 piece peeled ginger root (approximately 1/4" to 1/2")
1 piece cinnamon stick (approximately 1" long)
2 cups of water
Boil all ingredients 20 to 30 minutes with the lid on.
Add a pinch of black tea. Boil 5 more minutes.

Add 2 ounces of low fat or fat-free milk. (Add this only to amount you are going to be drinking that day.) Bring to a boil and immediately remove from heat.

Add honey to taste.

Enjoy!

If you did store some tea, just boil for several minutes, then add milk and serve.

The leftover ingredients from the first brew can be used a second time.

Chapter 9
"Your Body's Feedback System"
Behavioral Kinesiology

This section presents a unique system for assessing the impact of your inner attitudes and of all kinds of environmental stimuli (including food, people around you, even the paintings on a wall) on your health and well-being. Called Behavioral Kinesiology (BK), it was developed by John Diamond, M.D., and is outlined in his book, Your Body Doesn't Lie. I studied directly with Dr. Diamond for two years.

To understand the material in the chapter, you must try it on a partner. Seeing for yourself is the only way you will believe what is described here.

Kinesiology is the science of muscle checking. It is the body's feedback system. It allows us to easily see, immediately and directly, how everything around us and within us affects our strength, health, and ability to act. This chapter also includes BK techniques for regulating stress effects and strengthening your system.

After you have experienced a few of the checks, turn to the section on "How Kinesiology Works" for an explanation of how it works.

Finding Normal Resistance

1. You must have a partner to do this. Face your partner.
2. Your partner should raise one arm straight out, perpendicular to the body, thumb pointing towards floor. (It's as if you were in an old Western where the sheriff asks, "Which way did they go?" and the person points and says, "They went that-a-way.") The other arm is at your side.

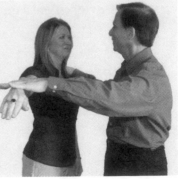

Step 2

3. Place one of your hands on your partner's extended arm, just above the wrist by the wrist bone. Place your other hand on partner's opposite shoulder.

4. Instruct your partner to resist as you push down, firmly, on the extended arm. You are not trying to force the arm all the way down; if the arm goes down more than a couple of inches, you were pressing too hard. You simply attempt to feel your partner's normal level of resistance. You should start firmly, not suddenly or with a jerk, and push for several seconds, then release.

The Power of the Mind

1. While your partner keeps her arm extended, have her think of an unhappy experience or someone she dislikes. Ask her to

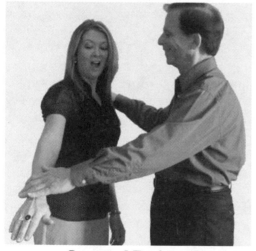

Lowered Resistance

tell you when she is focused on the thought. Tell her to keep thinking about it and to resist as you press on her arm. The arm will usually go down easily, even though your partner resists with all her might.

2. Wait several seconds; then tell your partner to resume the arm-up position while thinking of some enjoyable experience or someone she likes. Again, ask her to indicate when she has the thought focused, then tell her to resist as you push down on her arm. The arm will usually stay level and strong, even if you push harder than you did when you were finding her Normal Resistance.

3. Switch roles. Have your partner check you.

These are not tricks; the results are real and repeatable. In fact, I have taught hundreds of thousands of people to do it on each other at my keynotes and seminars.

The results have nothing to do with muscular strength, since you are checking only against the level of resistance the person has already demonstrated. You are also not attempting to push the person's arm all the way down. If the arm goes down more than a couple of inches, then you have pressed too hard. Simply, do it again with a little lighter pressure.

The thumb is turned down to make sure you are checking the same muscle each time: the deltoid. The deltoid runs from the front of the body right above the chest area, over the shoulder to the back. The deltoid muscle will either be capable of locking the arm into place, which means the body's life energy level is strong, or the arm will go down easily, which means the body's energy level

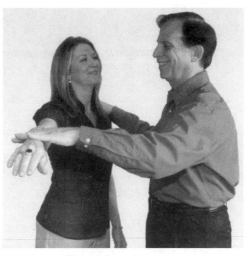

Checking Strong

has been weakened. The contrast is very easy to see and experience.

All of the muscle checks described in this chapter have been conducted with instruments that measure exactly how many pounds of pressure are being applied to the arm. Laboratory results prove to be identical to the results individuals get when muscle checking. When the person's arm goes down easily, it is not because you are suddenly pressing harder; it is because his or her life energy is weakened at that moment.

One research published in the journal *Perceptual and Motor Skills* (1999) was conducted with volunteers who had no experience with muscle checking. Each person said what their real name was and a false name. They also said that they were an American or a Russian (all the volunteers were American). The volunteers were muscle checked after making each statement. The results showed a dramatic consistence. On the false statements, the volunteer's arms went down 57% faster with 17% less pressure.

If you doing a number of checks on your partner or you are concerned that the person's arm is growing tired and will affect the results, feel free to have them switch to using their other arm to do the checking. Just be sure to check the "new" arm for Normal Resistance so you'll have a basis for comparison before going on to do the other checks in this section.

If you can't quite believe what's happening, check your partner as they think a variety of positive and negative thoughts. Have your partner check you while you think of a number of people that you like and dislike. If you check weak on a person you thought you sort of liked, you might want to reevaluate the relationship. Could the person be having a weakening impact on your energy level? Do you find yourself tired after being in their presence? Do you actually have mixed or ambivalent feelings towards the person? Is there an element of fear, envy, competition, or undermining going on?

Do you find it surprisingly easy to keep your arm steady while thinking of a pleasant scene or happy experience? Do you find that when you think of a painful or aggravating situation your arm goes down "like jelly?" It's almost as if your brain can't hear the command to "resist."

If you or a partner muscle checks strong on all the muscle checks in this section, including the tests that you would expect to generate a weakened response, please turn to the section of this chapter on "Strengthening the Thymus" (p. 124), and the last section (p. 125) for an explanation.

Positive Thoughts

In recent years, many books and articles have praised the idea of "positive thinking," including *The Secret* (which features a number of friends of mine—Jack Canfield, Marcy Shimoff, and Lisa Nichols). These works discuss the power of the mind over everyday life and the need to feed our minds positive thoughts as we feed our bodies healthful foods. They report extraordinary stories of success, achievement, happiness, and even "luck" resulting from positive thinking. Yet, for many people, this is just a concept, not something they have knowingly experienced or even believe. With kinesiology muscle checking, however, anyone can see the obvious, immediate impact of positive and negative thoughts on our bodies.

If you know someone who seems caught up in negative thoughts most of the time, look at that person's health. Does he become ill frequently? Does he have ulcers, arthritis, or high blood pressure? This person has fallen into a vicious cycle in which depressed or despairing thoughts weaken his body, which in turn becomes less able to cope with stress and negative thoughts!

When your mind is not concentrating on some specific task, does it tend to "wander" to whatever is most troubling or unsettled in your life? This is a habit many people have. I'm not referring to the act of consciously trying to think through a problem. I'm talking about a habit our minds have of settling on our own inadequacies, our dissatisfactions, our minor annoyances—and replaying them like a broken record. This is non-productive and weakening, and it wears away our problem-solving capacity! Next time you notice this habit, turn your mind deliberately to something happy—a memory, a plan, a dream, a hope, a good relationship, a work of art. Develop a new strengthening habit of letting your mind "wander" through positive territory

Optimists vs. Pessimists

A number of research studies have looked at optimism versus pessimism. One followed a class of Harvard graduates through their lives. The researchers found that the optimists outlived the pessimists by many years and that the optimists enjoyed life more. Another study looked at high blood pressure and found that optimists had three times less hypertension than pessimists. The most positive optimist had the lowest blood pressure level.

Optimists were 50 percent less likely to have cardiovascular disease; if an optimist did need bypass surgery, they were 50 percent less likely to have to return to the hospital after surgery.

Another study compared angry people with calm people. The researchers put cuts on all the volunteers' arms. They then tracked how long it took the cuts to heal. It took four times longer for the cuts on the arm of the angry person to heal versus the cuts on the calm person.

A negative work environment can impact your health, too. A 10-year study in Stockholm, Sweden observed the long-term health effects that a supervisor might have on his or her employees. Researchers tracked 3,000 men with an average age of 42 and better than average access to health care. Each participant rated their boss's behavior on ten measures, including statements such as "My boss gives me the information I need" and "I have sufficient power in relation to my responsibilities."

By the end of the study, 74 men had suffered heart attacks or other serious cardiac events. It turned out that the lower a boss's leadership score, the higher the worker's risk of a cardiac event. The chance of a heart attack also increased with the number of years of exposure to the same bad boss.

Such studies illustrate how positive or negative thinking can influence our longevity and our enjoyment of life.

Smiles and Frowns

As simple a stimulus as a smile or frown from another person can measurably affect your energy level. See for yourself:

1. Find your partner's Normal Resistance, as described on page 109.
2. Have your partner look at the photograph of a woman frowning. (Cover up the other photo of the woman smiling while you do this.) Place your hand on her extended arm,

just above the wrist, and push down firmly while she looks at the photo. Her arm should drop easily.

3. Now have your partner look at the photograph of the woman smiling. (Cover the frowning photo.) Have her extend her arm again; push down firmly on it as before. The arm should stay extended.

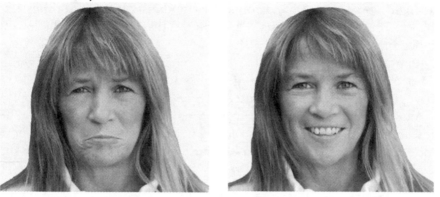

You can get the same results without photographs, simply by smiling or frowning at your partner as you check her. In fact, when doing any kinesiology checking, it is important to keep a "straight" or neutral expression on you face to avoid prejudicing the results. For many checks, the person being checked can also keep his eyes closed as "insurance" that what is in his hand or his thoughts is all that's being checked.

Next time you walk into a room and feel suddenly, unexpectedly uncomfortable, check people's expressions. You may be in a room full of frowning people!

Conversely, being around people who are smiling—or smiling yourself—is highly strengthening. You may have noticed that having a person in an office who smiles and is cheerful most of the time gives you a "lift," a sense of well-being. Even if you have no particular relationship with the person, and even if you have no "good reason" to feel good, you feel "lifted up" at least momentarily, every time that person smiles at you. Now you understand the reason: this person's smile and positive attitude have physically raised your energy level. A consistently cheerful, smiling person can thus tangibly help other people to get more done and to pursue their work more enthusiastically.

Foods

Foods also have a kinesiological effect on the body. Do this experiment:

1. Start with three identical envelopes. In one, place a teaspoon or packet of sugar; in the second, a teaspoon or packet of artificial sweetener; in the third, a couple of almonds or a spoonful of sesame seeds or sunflower seeds. Seal the envelopes; mix them up.
2. Check for Normal Resistance, as described on page 109.
3. Without telling your partner what substances are in the envelopes, give him one envelope to hold in the hand that's down at his side. Check his extended arm for resistance. Repeat with the other two envelopes, noting which check strong and which check weak. (You may want to number the envelopes and note the results on a piece of paper.)
4. Have your partner check you on each envelope.
5. Open all the envelopes and share the results.

The vast majority of people will check weak on the sugar and artificial sweetener, but strong on the almond, sunflower seed, or sesame seed. Research done on sugar and saccharin products correlates convincingly: These substances, and foods containing them, are unhealthy for most people. (See p. 78-84.) For confirmation, check again with each substance, one at a time, by placing them in the mouth.

As kinesiology demonstrates, the body knows instantly what is good or not good for it. As Dr. John Diamond has said, "The body is the best biochemist." Unfortunately, we have learned to consume foods that are terrible for our systems. As a matter of fact, the body can become addicted to foods that are not good for it, creating vicious cycles and much damage to your health. Sugar addiction, as discussed in pages 78-84, is an example.

Food Allergy Checking

Each individual's body chemistry and sensitivity (or allergic reaction) to various foods is different. One can have subtle "allergies" or toxic reactions that one is not aware of: A food may lower one's immunity to certain illnesses, cause depression or fatigue, headaches (as an example, a percentage of migraine sufferers are allergic to chocolate), stomach distress, etc. "Hyperactivity" in children is often an allergic reaction to sugar and chemical additives in foods (See pp. 78-84). Other common food allergies include milk, eggs, corn, and wheat.

Check for food allergies by placing a food (it can be placed in a napkin) in one hand, and checking the other arm for resistance. (Remember to check for Normal Resistance, with both hands empty, first.) When the arm goes down easily, it means the food being checked is not good for the person being checked. For confirmation, check again, with the food placed in the person's mouth as the mouth is more sensitive than the hand in detecting food allergies and sensitivities.

Eliminate foods that weaken you in these checks from your diet for several weeks. Then have yourself checked again; the results will probably be better because your body has had a rest from those foods. You may even be able to occasionally eat an offending food without seriously weakening your energies, but don't eat it more frequently than once every three or four days. Keep having your self checked. Some foods may remain too weakening for you to eat—ever.

I, personally, suffered for years from recurring gastroenteritis, which is excessive gas and belching. I tried many remedies including medical tests and treatments, special diets, and non-traditional healing methods such as acupuncture, massage, etc. No remedy eliminated the problem. When I learned about kinesiology, I had myself checked and discovered I checked weak on six or seven foods. I stopped eating those foods, and a problem I had for years was gone in four days.

If your children are eating (or demanding) a lot of sweets and other junk foods, check them. The technique will clearly show them how bad these products are for them. Their arm going down is very graphic to a child and may help you persuade them to eat more healthful foods. (Children, more than adults, tend to believe and follow through on what they can plainly see; after checking them, you may find them scoffing at the TV commercials that described Wonder (white) Bread "helping to build strong, healthy bodies.")

Vitamin Supplements

As I mentioned previously in the section on vitamins (p. 95), I believe vitamin supplements are necessary for us to achieve optimum health in our modern environment, even if we eat healthful, fresh foods. However, most people are confused about what supplements they should take, in what quantity, and whether the supplements should be natural or synthetic. Using kinesiology muscle checking to "ask" the body about its needs, all of these questions can be answered.

Make your mind "a blank." Have your partner check you for Normal Resistance. Hold the vitamin you are checking in your other hand, and have your partner check you again. If your arm goes down easily, it can mean one of several things:

The vitamin may be synthetic, and your system will function better on natural vitamins. Try checking yourself with a natural version versus the synthetic version of the vitamin.

The brand being checked may have an ingredient to which you are allergic. Check other brands of the same type and dosage of vitamins.

The dosage of this supplement may be too strong for your system. Check a smaller dosage.

Here is how to check for the quantity you should be taking. Start with a vitamin on which you've already checked strong. Add one more of that vitamin to your hand and check again. Keep adding more tablets or capsules, and check until your arm checks weak. At that point, you've exceeded your maximum dosage. Reduce the number of pills or capsules until you are checking very strong again. That is your maximum daily dosage.

Check yourself again, periodically (every few months or when your life has changed greatly), on all the supplements you routinely take. One's needs may change over time, particularly at times of increased emotional or physical stress, when the body needs many more nutrients to defend itself against illness and other stress effects.

I did an interesting "in the blind" experiment using vitamins with a medical doctor friend and a group of other doctors. My friend had checked strong on one supplement, weak on another. We wrapped each supplement individually in paper so no one could tell them apart. A third person, a nuclear physicist, mixed them up, out of our view. The doctor selected one of the wrapped packages in his hand and held it behind his back. I turned around, faced him, and checked his extended arm. If he checked strong, I said he was holding Supplement X, and if he checked weak, I named Supplement Y. The physicist verified and recorded the results.

I was correct eighteen out of twenty times, a 90 percent accuracy rate. Participants and observer doctors concluded that something significant had occurred, though they were at a loss to explain it through their usual medical or scientific understanding.

Checking Your Workplace

Remember how much a simple smile or frown could affect your energy level? Since we are taught to suppress our emotions, particularly at work, it's likely that you are having negative (and positive) reactions to all sorts of things at work without being aware of them or taking them seriously. Kinesiology checking is an excellent way to find out which people, events, and parts of your physical environment at work are strengthening you and which ones are weakening you and increasing your stress.

Have someone check you as you think about each of your coworkers, superiors, subordinates, and frequent business contacts, one at a time.

How do you spend your time at work? Have yourself checked while thinking about each of your major tasks.

Besides rearranging your work relationships and your duties as much as possible to emphasize the ones that strengthen you the most, there are remedies to counteract the weakening effect of aspects of your work that are negative to you (see p. 120). If too many aspects of your work environment check negative and you can't make changes, you might want to consider a career or workplace change.

You can also check elements in your physical environment—your decor, paintings, colors, wall paints, etc.—just by looking at or touching the thing you're interested in, while your partner checks your arm for resistance.

The next two sections deal with environmental aspects that can have a profound impact on workplace well-being: lighting and music.

Fluorescent Lights

Check your partner for Normal Resistance (see p. 103). Then find a fluorescent light. Have your partner look directly at it while you check her arm. She will check weak.

What your partner has experienced is the effect of "cool white" fluorescent tubes, which comprises most of the fluorescent lighting used in offices. The book *Health and Light*, by John Ott, documents the ways in which the combination of light waves in "cool white" fluorescents adversely affects our systems. Office workers report feelings of sleepiness, despair, nervousness, irritability, nausea, and dizziness—all of which disappear when lighting is changed to incandescent or a special type of "full-spectrum" fluorescent bulb.

Ott was the filmmaker who produced the original Walt Disney time-lapse films of flowers blooming very quickly. He shot one frame every few minutes over a period of days; when the film was sped up, the flowers unfolded gracefully before the viewer's eyes. Ott discovered that different colors of light affect plants in different ways. Some colors or combinations are beneficial; others are deleterious.

Ott then turned to researching the effects of light on humans. He reported a variety of startling improvements that occur when full-spectrum fluorescent lights are introduced into a work situation. Industries have experienced a 25 percent increase in productivity. In colleges, students' abilities to concentrate and to retain information have risen measurably; and in grammar schools, children who have been hyperactive have suddenly become calm and cooperative when the lighting is changed.

To illustrate the impact on children, there is a charter school in Maitland, Florida called Summit Charter School. Its student body is composed of grammar school level kids who all suffer from a variety of learning disabilities and difficulties. The principal, Alan Smolowe decided to compare the school's cool white tubes with the full spectrum tubes. Teachers keep records on the for six weeks while they were under the cool white tubes tracking things like behavior, attention, and concentration. A the end of six weeks, they replaced the cold white ith ectrum tubes and monitored the same asp The teachers and the principal were astonished by the leveive changes in the kids. One teacher, in a gloohe positive impact of the frum lighting, added thiIf mpt to take thee tubes out of my classroom, I will fight you, and I will change the lock on my door"How's that for an impact!

Millions suffer from seasonal depression, called Seasonal Affective Disorder (SAD), in fall and winter when days shorten. When morning comes, their bodies fail to shut off the production of melatonin. Research shows that the body's internal clock is most sensitive to the blue portion of the light spectrum, which is more effective than other light in halting production of melatonin and resetting the body's clock.

The lack of quality light which also results in a low level of serotonin affects many people, both female and male. When serotonin is high, we feel good and are more relaxed and focused. Melatonin, which helps us sleep deeply at night, is produced by the brain's pineal gland when we're in the dark or dim light.

Bright light, specifically blue wavelengths, suppresses melatonin and raises serotonin, enabling us to function at a more optimal level—just what we want during the day. But working in an office all day under traditional fluorescent lighting does not provide the benefits our bodies need from daylight. Full spectrum light provides the appropriate blue-white light, the closest to natural sunlight, suppressing melatonin and helping us wake up and be more alert and yet calm.

Research has found there are dramatic health benefits to be gained with full spectrum light that includes trace amounts of ultraviolet in the same proportion that the sun emits. But don't worry—the ultraviolet light is safe, not at the levels used in tanning beds.

Additional researchd the importance of Scientists at Brown University have discovered a third type of photoreceptor cell in the eye. Urelated to the rods and cones in our eye,these cells are directly connected to the brain's hypothalamus. The hypothalamus, together with the pituitary gland, controls your body clock, hormones and moods. It also controls the dilation of your irises and helps you cus without eye. This newly dor cell "ses" only one color of light: sky blue! True full pectrum lghting pces color in this sky-blue wavelength, which furthr supports their benefits.

Most people spend at least eight hours a day working, studying, or traveling under "cool white" fluorescent bulbs. It's hard to tell how much fatigue, boredom, and illness—on and off the job—result from the wrong type of lighting.

Check the lighting you are using in your home, too. Most people are exchanging their incandescent bulbs for compact fluorescent lighting. While ompact fuorescent lghts (CFLs) offer great energy savings, they present the same problems workers have been experiencing in offices. Most CLFs sold today have a high level of yellow in them, which sunlight doesn't have. Instead, manufacturers mask the yellow. You want to choose a bulb that allows the light emanating from it to be full spectrum.

JTV Energy Lights offers true full-spectrum lights. All of their fluorescent tubes operate in regular fluorescent fixtures. They have tubes, bulbs, , and CFLs hat simulate the full color and ultraviolet spectrum of daylight. You can find them online at www.JTV-Energy-Lights.com.

Changing the lighting in homes, schools, offices, factories, and public places to fullspectrum lighting may be one of the most effective single things you can do to reduce stress in these difficult times. People who work at the Greater Lansing Association of Realtors actually call their full spectrum tubes their "happy lights!"

Music

Music, like everything else in the environment, can be beneficial or detrimental to us. Dr. John Diamond has found that much of hard rock music weakens the body's energy system. According to him, the weakening effect seems to be caused by a certain beat that is common in this kind of rock music, a rhythm of "da-da-DA," which repeats in such a way that the song almost seems to stop momentarily after each measure (after each "DA"). (In poetry, this is known as an anapestic beat.)

Dr. Diamond has found correlations between this type of sound and a phenomenon called "switching" in which the left side and right side of the brain cease working together in balance. Many innocuous everyday activities can cause "switching," as Diamond explains in his book Your Body Doesn't Lie. When switching has occurred, one side of the brain is working too hard. Thinking or solving problems becomes more difficult, and the person experiences increased stress. Since this is a state some people experience a lot, they don't notice these effects consciously, except for a vague sense of confusion, discomfort, or fatigue. The feeling may be "There's too much going on here," or "I have more demands on me than I can deal with."

Since not all rock music weakens us, check it for yourself. Have a partner check you for Normal Resistance, then check again while you're listening to a particular song. You can check everything on your mp3 or iPod this way to see which music actually strengthens you, which is neutral to you, and which music weakens you. If music is played in your workplace, check some of the people there to see how it is affecting them. Perhaps you can change the music, or have it changed, to something that has a strengthening effect, check it and see.

Dr. Diamond cites the following example in Your Body Doesn't Lie:

"One factory in particular, a manufacturing and repair plant for sophisticated electronic equipment, where concentration and clear-headedness are essential, was playing a great deal of rock on its continual music broadcast system. It was recommended that this be eliminated. The management changed to different music and found to their delight an immediate increase in productivity and an equally pleasing decrease in errors, even though the employees were quite vocal about their dissatisfaction at having their favorite music removed."

This anecdote illustrates the fact that people can become addicted to music that is unhealthy, just as we can become addicted to unhealthy foods. From birth, if you are exposed to things that are unhealthy or stressful to your body, you can become accustomed to the stresses and this state of disease You can actually get to the point that you crave this negative stimuli as much or more than you would crave positive stimuli.

Yet, people who investigate what would be healthy for them and discipline themselves to eat healthy foods, do the right activity, or use appropriate vitamin supplements generally find after a period of time that they feel better than they have ever felt in their lives. Their bodies become less confused and more instinctively sensitive to anything unhealthy. They find they can "taste" artificial additives or colorings in foods; they feel uncomfortable or ill when they eat or drink something unhealthy; and when something in the environment lowers their energy level or dampens their spirits, they generally notice it immediately because of the contrast with their now-typical sense of well-being.

An example would be a smoker who has no awareness of the intense odor of tobacco smoke. When the person quits smoking, their sense of smell becomes hyper-aware when tobacco smoke is in their environment.

If you own or manage a business and you want to change the music, the food served in the lunchroom, or anything else that directly affects employees, the best procedure is to meet with your employees, explain the change and discuss and the expected benefits, have them experience the kinesiology checking, and make the change on a trial basis. People are much more likely to cooperate with such an approach than when changes are forced on them, even "for their own good."

Recently, some composers have begun to use kinesiology checking to make sure their music is strengthening. One such composer is Steven Halpern, Ph.D. He describes as "anti-frantic" the series of compositions he designed especially to be relaxing and energizing. He has also developed a music series with subliminal messages. Some of these CD titles are:

Achieving Your Ideal Weight	Stop Smoking
Accelerated Learning	Radiant Health and Well-being
Creativity	Enhancing Self-Esteem
Enhancing Success	Accelerated Self-Healing
Effortless Relaxation	Attracting Prosperity
Sleep Soundly	

I have produced several business subliminal CDs with Steven, including Success For Sales People and Success For Managers. Find his music online at www.Teplitz.com.

Let me share some stories about the impact of Halpern's music. The first two involve Connections by Steven and Paul Horn. I worked with a company that decided to play Connections as hold music on their phone system. An irate client called and was put on hold by a customer service representative. It took over two minutes for the customer service rep to pick up the line again. Amazingly, the client was no longer angry! Just listening to Connections calmed him down. It actually became company policy to put an irate customer on hold for two minutes.

Another story is about the owner of a restaurant who saw me demonstrate the positive impact of Connections at my seminar. He decided to do an experiment, and he played it in his restaurant every hour on the hour for thirty minutes. In that half-hour period, he discovered that check amounts went up, tips went up, and complaints went down.

A third story is about the subliminal CD by Halpern called Accelerating Learning. I gave this CD to my stepson, Adam, to use when he went to college. He and his girlfriend, Eileen, played it whenever they studied. After two years, their relationship ended. Eileen called me to say Adam got "custody" of the Accelerating Learning CD and asked if I could send her a copy of her own (which I did).

The final story, I was visiting a friend to deliver a copy of the Accelerating Learning CD for her son. At the time he was studying math. He took the CD and went into his room to continue studying. Five minutes later he comes out and says, "I put on the music and all of a sudden the math made sense."

The Meridian Check

Acupuncture asserts that the body has specific meridians or energy pathways that connect points related mostly to the body's organs. Understanding and using these energetic pathways has contributed to the remarkable success of acupuncture in curing a variety of mental and physical disturbances and in improving one's health. Even Western medical scientists have identified distinct electrical sites on the body that coincide with the main acupuncture points on a meridian. (See also the chapter on Shiatsu, p. 13.)

We can use these meridians to align the body's energetic system and reduce stress.

1. Check for Normal Resistance (See p. 103). While your partner keeps the position, arm extended, use one of your hands to trace a straight line, from your partner's eye to his foot without touching his body.
2. Immediately check the resistance in your partner's arm by telling him to resist as you push down. The arm will usually go down much more easily than normal. Surprised?
3. Have your partner extend his arm again. This time, trace a line along the body from your partner's foot to the eye, without touching him.

4. Immediately check your partner's ability to resist. You will find your partner staying strong again.
5. Switch and have your partner check you.

Almost everyone checks weak when a hand is run from the eye to the foot and strong when they trace the line from the foot to the eye.

There are fourteen main meridians on the body, and they run in specific pathways. Running from the eye to the foot and back up again impacts the stomach meridian.

Let's check another meridian called the spleen meridian. Check for Normal Resistance (see p. 103). Now, with your hand at your partner's waist level (where she would wear a belt), trace a line—without touching her body—from her arm to her belly button. Do it just one time. Now, immediately check her resistance. As you push on the extended arm, it should go down easily.

One common activity that consistently cuts the spleen meridian is ironing clothes. The repetitive back-and-forth motion at the waistline breaks the energy flow of the spleen meridian. No wonder ironing is so fatiguing!

To re-strengthen the spleen meridian, lightly massage the area you traced with your hand, moving from the side to the belly button. You must actually touch the person this time. Immediately re-check your partner's resistance. The extended arm will usually stay firm.

How Kinesiology Works

Now that you've had several experiences of the Kinesiology Muscle Checking, let me give you an understanding of how it works. One of your first questions might be: How can these meridians be affected when our bodies are not even touched?

One explanation is found in research developed in the 1940s in Bulgaria called Kirlian photography. A person places their finger on an electrical plate, and a slight electrical charge is run through the plate. Using special photographic equipment, the photographer is able to capture the image of a band of light with colors in it, sometimes several inches deep, which extends out from the finger. Research has led Kirlian photographers to conclude that the light and color comprise an energy band emanating from the body, which is as individual as a fingerprint.

In fact, any person, animal, plant, or other living thing photographed in this manner will reveal such an aura. Could this simply be a picture of the electricity being transmitted through the object or body? No, because each person's aura is different and because the aura changes radically, depending on what the person is doing, thinking, feeling, and the state of the person's health at the time of the photograph. Significantly, inanimate objects or once-living things that have been dead longer than a few hours do not show up in Kirlian photographs. Even metals that are electrical conductors do not produce Kirlian images.

Researchers are compiling data that correlate changes in the color and shape of the energy field with specific physical and psychological states (such as cancer, depression, etc.), suggesting that Kirlian photography has the potential to be used as a medical diagnostic tool.

I have experienced aura photography that is similar to Kirlian photography. I placed my hand on a special plate that records the energy charge from the hand. A video monitor displayed my image and the various colors in the surrounding energy band. I experimented with changing my thoughts from positive to negative, and was actually able to see the colors and shape of the energy band change as the energy of my thoughts changed.

These technologies reveal tangible, physical energy body that emanating from every living thing. The mild electrical charge illuminates this normally invisible energy the way a sunbeam illuminates tiny dust particles that are normally invisible in the air. We can see that living things give off unique, perceivable energy that reacts to internal and external stimuli.

Our brains make billions of unconscious calculations and translations every day to tell us what is going on around us; these calculations include information from our "sixth sense" (perceptions of the energy and emotions of other people and things around us), in addition to information from our eyes, ears, nose, taste, and the conscious aspects of touch. You may also be aware of this "sixth sense" when you suddenly "look up" or look around just in time to avoid a collision or mishap of some sort. What probably has happened is that your energy field and the energy field of whatever you were about to collide with started to make contact. The fields "bumped" first, and you sensed that interaction.

Perhaps our energy fields perceive and "read" the fact that there is sugar or some weakening substance in an envelope we're holding, just as our eyes perceive and our brains interpret that we are seeing a "book," a "desk," or a "car."

Your energy field is directly affected by everything happening, inside and outside you. It appears that, properly understood, a person's energy field is a detailed picture of everything the person is experiencing at a given moment—physical, mental, emotional, spiritual.

Evidence shows that touching the energy field can have the same effects as touching the person's body directly. This is why you can "cut" your partner's meridian just by running your hand from your partner's eye to the foot. The process is similar to what happens when a station is coming in quite clearly on your car radio and, as you drive along, a second station begins to interfere. One radio frequency is interfering with another. Another analogous situation is created by placing a magnet near an electrical wire. The magnet will measurably interfere with the flow of current, even though the magnet is not touching the wire.

The impact on a meridian is the same: you can't see it, but the body knows it immediately.

A friend of mine applied this in his weightlifting. Recall that the stomach meridian runs from each foot to the eye above it, and that moving a hand in this direction is strengthening. In his customary workout, this man had always lifted and lowered barbells very close to his body. I explained to him that every time he lifted the barbells up he was strengthening this meridian, but that every time he lowered them, he was weakening himself. I actually did the muscle checking on him, so he got to experience what I was saying. He immediately modified his lifting, keeping the barbells close to his body on the upstroke from the foot to over the head. Before he lowered the barbell, he moved his hands out, so that his hands were away from his body. He reported an immediate improvement: he was able to exercise longer and lift more weight. He even felt that his workout became easier.

Our meridians may be cut frequently during the day in normal interactions. When you pass someone in the hallway or on an elevator, one of you may move your arm in such a way that it cuts the other's spleen meridian. Normally, the body will readjust the energy imbalance. (See section on The Role of the Thymus, page 120.) However, if you are doing repetitive activities such as typing on your computer all day long, it can contribute to an accumulation of stresses that leaves the body fatigued by the end of the day.

Meridian Strengthening Breaks

One way to prevent fatigue is to take several "meridian strengthening breaks" throughout the day. Simply trace the line from one foot to the eye several times during the day. Do it for a few days and see if you feel less tired at the end of the day.

You can also rub your hand along the spleen meridian line from your arm to your belly button as another way to give yourself a strengthening break.

Changing Your Energy: Overcoming Stress

There are several techniques you can use to alter the way in which stress affects you. Besides meditation, deep breathing, and yoga described in earlier chapters, there are exercises and habits discovered through kinesiological research that specifically strengthen and balance our energy systems. Among them are the ones I've already shared with you—meridian strengthening, turning your mind to positive thoughts, and smiling. (Positive thinking and smiling are not accomplished by repressing or ignoring incidents that bother you and the feelings that follow. Rather, negative feelings should be faced, examined, understood, and left behind. Though this may not be easy, several of the techniques in this section of the book will help. I will elaborate on this later in the chapter.)

The Energy Button

First, do the following check. Later, I'll explain what occurred. You'll need a packet of sugar.

1. Check your partner for Normal Resistance, as described on page 103.
2. Give her the packet of sugar to hold as you check her arm again. It should go down easily.
3. Tell your partner to place her tongue gently against the roof of her mouth, about 1/4 inch behind the front teeth.
4. Have her keep her tongue up while she holds the sugar and you check her again.

What happened? Almost everyone's arm will stay up as long as the tongue is "up" against the roof of the mouth. As soon as the tongue is lowered, the negative effects of the sugar will return. The tongue, in that position at the roof of the mouth, acts as an energy button or switch.

Placing the tongue up is analogous to turning on a light switch. Until the light switch touches the contact point, electricity will not flow through the system. Similarly, placing the tongue at the roof of the mouth closes the body's internal circuitry, allowing the energy to flow. In a sense, it is turning on our internal light switch.

Developing the habit of keeping the tongue at the roof of the mouth about 1/4 inch behind the front teeth will negate the effects of stress. It's best to keep the tongue in this position at all times, except when you are talking or eating. After reminding yourself a number of times to keep the tongue up, you will find that "up" becomes its natural resting place, without conscious thought on your part. Many people notice that after they've done this for a few days, their tongues habitually rest in the "up" position, and keeping the tongue down becomes an effort!

When your tongue is up, your meridians will not be weakened in the ways I've previously described.

Keeping the tongue to the roof of the mouth can be noticeably beneficial in sports or in any physical activity. This is partly because different kinds of body movement—including specific movements used in sports—can strengthen or weaken our energy systems. As an example, do this experiment:

1. Check your partner for Normal Resistance, as described on page 103.
2. Have your partner do three golf swings or three jumping jacks.
3. Now check his ability to resist. You'll find he checks weak.

Golfers almost always take practice swings before hitting the ball. This movement of the swing is actually affecting the spleen meridian and creating a weakening effect on the golfer's body. Read on to find out what you can do to prevent this energy drain.

Tennis players face a similar problem with backhand strokes. The backhand movement weakens the player's energy level because it causes "switching"—a distortion of the communication between the left and right hemispheres of the brain.

Switching produces an unconscious confusion in the body, stress, and a weakening of energy. We have already mentioned that it can be triggered by some types of hard rock music (p. 114). Among the other body movements that can "switch" a person are common jumping jacks, in which the arm and leg movements mirror each other exactly. (This is a "homolateral" movement.) A different type of jumping jack, in which arms are together while legs are apart, and vice versa, does not switch our brain hemispheres and, thus, is not weakening. This movement is a "hetero-lateral" movement similar to walking when you are swinging your opposite arm in sync with your opposite leg.

Recheck your partner on the three golf swings or three homolateral jumping jacks; but this time, have him put his tongue to the roof of his mouth while he's doing the movements. This time, his resistance will stay strong. The tongue on our "energy light switch" is allowing the body to maintain its energy level and is preventing the weakening effects of these body motions. (If you are wondering if the strengthening effect could be "the power of suggestion," do a set of these checks without telling your partner what the tongue position is supposed to do.)

Many golfers who have attended my business seminars have played a round of golf while keeping their tongue up. They told me that they were consistently driving the ball 25 to 35 yards farther. Recently, one golfer reported he had taken sixteen strokes off his game!

I shared the concept of the energy button with a bicycle racer, who was skeptical about its effectiveness. Not long after, he was in a bike race and found himself becoming tired. He decided to use the tongue-up technique. He immediately regained his energy and went on to win the race.

A middle-aged runner who competes in five-mile races told me he noticed a marked improvement in his racing time after he started keeping his tongue up during the entire race.

The Role of the Thymus Gland

Certainly the stronger your energy system is, the better you will be able to deal with any stress aggravations that arise. The thymus gland plays a central role in regulating our personal energy system. Once thought by the medical profession to have no function in adults, the thymus is now known as the body's center of immunity and resistance. It "trains" lymphocytes—white blood cells that fight infection—to do their job, and it sends out hormones to help direct lymphocyte activity throughout the body. It also produces T-cells and B-cells that are of major importance to the functioning of our immune system.

Thymus activity is also central to the theory of cancer developed by Australian Nobel Prize winner Sir MacFarlane Burnet. He has stated that, of the billions of new cells produced in the body each day, some will always be abnormal. Thymus-derived lymphocytes (T-cells) can recognize and destroy these abnormal cells. But, if T-cells are not activated by the thymus hormone, some abnormal cells may survive, lodge themselves somewhere in the body, and grow into cancer. Thus, according to Burnet, the thymus gland is critical to cancer prevention.

This theory is supported by the fact that cancer occurrence increases with age. Thymus activity in mammals decreases with age. (The antibody response of elderly mice is only about five percent that of young mice, Dr. Diamond reports.)

Each new piece of research on the thymus reveals it to be more important than the last. Research findings have shown that the thymus gland is not only intimately involved with the immunological system, but also regulates the flow of energy throughout the body from moment to moment. It is the job of the thymus to both defend the body from illness and to repair (as best it can) the effects of stress.

Thus, when a meridian is "cut," the thymus will readjust the energy flow back to that meridian. By the end of the day, due to ongoing stress and fatigue, the readjustment process is taking longer and longer, and we are feeling more and more tired.

Strengthening the Thymus

The thymus gland is located about where the second button on a shirt would be located, in the center of the chest just below the collarbone. It's an inch or so below the hollow at the base of the throat. You will feel a slight bump, hill, or protrusion there; that's the thymus.

Tapping or thumping on this spot has a very beneficial effect on the entire body. Tapping the thymus immediately energizes the entire energy system and will rapidly cancel out most stress effects. Tap the spot rapidly with your fingertips ten to fifteen times. Doing this routinely, five or six times a day, will assist you in successfully handling short-term stress. The length of time during which the thymus will stay strong varies with the person and the types of stressful situations one encounters. The more stressful the environment, the less time the benefit lasts.

To check the strength of your thymus, place two or three fingers on the thymus spot, touching the skin. Have someone check your other arm for resistance. If you check weak, tap or thump the thymus spot hard ten to fifteen times. Then have your arm checked again while your fingers are in place. Your arm will not budge and will feel stronger.

Special objects and music can have the same stimulating effect on the thymus. If you look at the object or listen to the song and your arm stays strong when you put your fingers on the thymus, then you have discovered something that is actually energizing your system. If you find a picture that does this, place it on your desk and keep glancing at it over the course of a day. Looking at this picture is giving your stress resistance equipment a boost.

What If You Check Strong on Everything?

Occasionally, you may find a person who checks strong on everything. This person's arm will not check weak with sugar, saccharin, fluorescent lights, frowns, touching the thymus, or anything. This means that the person's life energy is not being affected by the stresses around her. They comprise less than 5 percent of the population. In an audience of several hundred people, I generally find only one or two people in this group. It is a good place for a person to be. It doesn't mean the person never feels bad about anything; it just means that her body, thymus, and energy system are dealing with these feelings without being weakened. It simply takes a lot more stress to blow this person's energy circuits.

Another possibility is that the person is what I call a "pseudo five-percenter." Adrenaline being secreted by the body is keeping her arm up. Adrenaline is the body's flight-or-fight response—as a survival mechanism it overrides the entire circuitry of the body. In fact, the person will initially muscle check like a five-percenter, as her arm will stay up when you check the thymus gland.

The way to determine if the person is a true five-percenter or a pseudo five-percenter is to have her tap the outer sides of her hands together (the side you use in a karate chop). Tap them together 35 to 45 times. When she places her fingers back on the thymus gland and the arm comes down, it means she is a pseudo five-percenter. Tapping shuts off the adrenal glands secretions, so you can now muscle check the person with confidence.

If, after tapping the sides of the hands together, the person's arm still stays up when she put her fingers on the thymus gland, you have further confirmation that the person is a true five-percenter, and you cannot do the muscle checking on her.

Becoming a true five-percenter is a trait that we can develop. By following the techniques laid out in this book, cleaning up you diet, doing meditation, and following an exercise program, you have the potential of becoming high energy, all the time.

Handling Emotional Issues

Earlier in the chapter, you learned about the visceral impacts of positive and negative thoughts and feelings. Negative thoughts diminish a person's strength, energy level, and stress resistance. In a challenging economy, it can be difficult to keep your thoughts upbeat. Paradoxically, focusing on negative thoughts makes a person less capable of handling negative situations, touchy issues, or upsetting stressful events.

The act of repressing or ignoring negative feelings without understanding them can contribute to stress. Repression, or denying one's own truth, takes tremendous amounts of energy. And the repressed feelings may still weaken you because they are stored somewhere in your mind.

While it's best to recognize, accept, and understand these feelings and then let them go, calmly and cheerfully, it is difficult to do. You may experience your mind continually bringing up the negative feelings. Even though you take action on the situation that caused the feelings in the first place, you may continue to have these negative feelings interrupting your thoughts.

Many of the relaxation techniques in this book—meditation, yoga, and deep breathing—will relieve much of the intensity of these feelings. Here's another technique that will allow you to feel that you have taken "a step back" from the negative feeling and diminished or even gotten rid of the negative energy attached to those thoughts so that the feeling loses its impact on you.

While you will initially perform this technique with a partner, once you've learned it, you can do the technique by yourself to get rid of the negative energy. This comes from the book *Touch for Health* by John Thie, D.C.

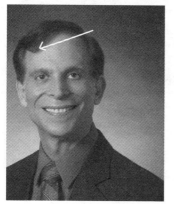

Frontal Lobes

1. Check your partner for Normal Resistance. Now have your partner think of something negative and stressful. Check her extended arm; it will go down easily.

2. Have your partner find the middle of her eyebrows. Have her then move her three middle fingers up to the middle of her forehead where the head begins to curve: the frontal lobe of the brain. Have your partner think about and visualize the negative situation in as much detail as possible.

3. While she is holding this position she may find the negative thoughts fading away, her mind wandering off, other unrelated thoughts happening. When any of these things occur, ask her to start viewing the situation positively.

4. She should continue to gently touch the forehead points for up to five minutes.

5. You'll know the negative energy has been eliminated from the thought when you recheck your partner's extended arm while she thinks of the same situation and her arm stays strong.

With the charge taken off the thought, it will be easier for her to confront and deal effectively with the situation. Will this negative thought be gone forever? The answer is: maybe yes and maybe no. In most cases, it will be gone; however, if it comes back, simply hold the points on the forehead again for a few more minutes.

Chapter 10
Sex and Relaxation

In difficult and stressful times, there may be no more effective, affordable, and...well, fun strategy to reduce stress than sex! While stress can contribute to a low level of desire, sex can be the solution! Research suggests that sexual activity reduces stress levels and improves your mood. And if your mood improves, you'll want to have more sex, so you increase the benefits even more. Sexual activity can help to reduce blood pressure and to prevent a sharp rise when you're experiencing a stressful event.

In one study of middle-aged women, intimate activity with a partner reduced the woman's stress and boosted her mood the next day. Another study of participants' blood pressure before a stressful event found that those who had recently had intercourse tended to have either lower baseline blood pressure levels, less of an increase in blood pressure when under stress, or both.

Sex provides specific stress-management benefits. The deep breathing involved relaxes the body, oxygenates the blood, and reduces stress levels. The touch involved provides us a much-needed boost to our emotional health. Endorphins and other hormones that boost mood are released. And the emotional intimacy in sex with a partner supports the need for a strong social support network.

Speaking of social networks, research is also demonstrating the value of personal relationships beyond intimate ones. One study demonstrated that the connection between people is a vibratory one. Consider a tuning fork: when you strike it, it begins to vibrate. If that tuning fork is next to another tuning fork of the same frequency, it will also vibrate. A study conducted by Russek and Schwartz had two people wired with EKGs and EEGs sitting in a room without contact of any kind. The researchers discovered three things:

1. Each person's heart was transmitting energy to his or her brain.
2. One person's heart was exchanging energy with the other person's brain.
3. Both people's hearts were also exchanging energy.

When we feel attracted to someone, we may actually be experiencing a connection with the other person on more levels than we ever realized before.

Here's another tip to increase a sense of connection and develop intimacy. Scientists using magnetic resonance imaging discovered that the pleasure centers of the brain respond much more strongly to unexpected stimuli than to expected, pleasurable ones. To me, this means in intimate relationships when you do the unexpected, your loved one will be much more excited than when you do the expected. 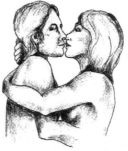 So keep those flowers, cards, letters, and kisses coming, but do them when they are unexpected.

Besides the "regular" reasons for having a sexual relationship, there's a heart-related reason as well. Research on the lives of heart attack patients showed that half of the victims have one thing in common. They did not have any kind of sexual activity for the entire year preceding the heart attack. Need I say more?

Finally for women, don't let physical discomforts when having sex stop the intimacy and the benefits of the experience. Postmenopausal women who are sexually active rarely hear their doctors asking about sexual problems like pain and dryness. Less than nine percent of doctors ask adult women about these issues. Since your doctor won't raise the subject, you need to get over your embarrassment and tell your doctor if you are having these or other sexual issues.

Sex can be both relaxing and energizing if a particular method called tantric yoga is followed.

Tantric yoga is an ancient Eastern technique. One of the main characteristics is that the sex act is performed without the male having an ejaculation. This means that lovemaking can go on for long periods of time. In "Western" style sex, the act is over once the male has ejaculated. He has lost the energy to continue. Without an ejaculation, the male can continue to relate while the energy level continues to build. The result will be an increase in the energy both partners feel much more intensely than during "regular" sex.

Relaxation also occurs because the physical movements are much slower in tantric yoga. Instead of looking for peaks of excitement through rapid movements, the partners are seeking valleys of relaxation through slower and easier movements. There is no rush to orgasm. You can imagine it as strolling through a beautiful meadow on a Sunday afternoon.

For the woman, enjoyment is actually increased because the length of time and the stimulation is increased. The woman can actually have as many orgasms as she desires. The orgasms the woman experiences increase the energy level of both partners. The man may find himself having orgasms—release of tension through his entire body—without ejaculating. The partners will not tire, or will be very slow to tire, because there is no tension and pushing for these experiences. It is more like letting a wave wash over you.

The end results are deeply relaxing and energizing.

A man who ordinarily rolls over and goes to sleep after sex will find he can instead continue to be active and relate to the woman. Even a man who doesn't habitually fall asleep will find he has more energy than he would usually after sex.

Another benefit is that it lets each partner feel and experience the other more fully. Ordinarily, when one is enjoying sex, one tends to be conscious of the feelings in one's own body. With tantric yoga, the length of the act and the slowness allow each partner to experience what the other is feeling...to really sense what is happening in the other's body. It is a very conscious sort of merging.

Tantric yoga should be done with a partner you care about. There must be increased communication between the partners. You need to be clear with each other on expectations and on the actual movements which are taking place—how does this feel...would something else be better...and so on. This results in the development of a deeper rapport and understanding between the partners.

Success in tantric yoga depends greatly on the male's attitude. He must change his focus from intense movement to reach orgasm to one of slowing and lengthening the sex act. Reducing the competitive attitude many men bring to sex is an important step in allowing the relaxation from tantric yoga to flow in. The woman, too, must measure "success" differently, as it is not having the man achieve orgasm.

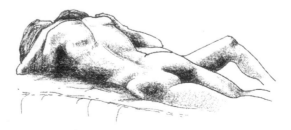

Here are some guidelines that will aid in developing tantric yoga for yourself and your partner:

1. Keep breathing. Instead of "panting," you take long, deep breaths that fill your body. As I discussed in the breathing section (pp. 9), deep breathing keeps you relaxed and keeps you from tensing your muscles. By continuing to breathe, you will begin to experience the valleys of relaxation of tantric yoga.

2. Keep the movement slow. Movement is necessary for the man to maintain an erection; however, too much movement can stimulate an ejaculation. (It's all right for the man to ejaculate once every few times he does tantric yoga.)

3. Movement doesn't have to be constant. It's okay to stop and rest. If the man is feeling too stimulated, just rest in the position you're both in at that moment.

4. Explore all kinds of movements. Touch, massage, caress…do anything that feels pleasurable.

5. After becoming familiar with the technique, some couples have found they enjoy having discussions or even reading to each other during tantric yoga.

6. Change positions. Avoid positions in which the man is receiving a lot of stimulation; for example, with the man on top of the woman. Since you will be communicating throughout the experience, talk about which positions feel helpful and which do not. Be willing to experiment.

Don't be upset if you are not completely successful the first times you try tantric yoga. It takes practice and requires a period of adjustment to become adept at it and to feel all the benefits. The result, though, will be rewarding as you open yourself to new vistas in your sexual relationships and new avenues of relaxation in your life.

Index

This index will guide you to some, but not necessarily all, of the appropriate techniques for relieving pains and strengthening, relaxing, and toning various parts of the body. If one method doesn't suit you, try another. However, don't try any exercise or treatment in a chapter until you've read the introduction to that chapter at least once. The index also includes various subjects that are discussed or mentioned in the book.

Executives and Associations Applaud Jerry Teplitz's Programs:

"What can I say...? You were a smash! We have never had a turnout for an education session like we did for yours. They all loved it! You were one of the high points of our convention."
> Peggie Hagan, Convention Manager, NATIONAL UTILITY
> CONTRACTORS ASSOCIATION

"I received considerable insight into methods of relieving stress. Fatigue is well accepted as a cause of poor decisions and aircraft accidents. Your presentation would seem a natural for airlines and other aviation organizations."
William H. Cox, Editor, Corporate Flight Magazine

"You could have heard a pin drop. You had our Annual Business and Management Meeting participants so entranced! As the highest rated speaker of our meeting, it's a pleasure to send our sincere thanks for a terrific job."
> Barbara Klemm, Director of Conferences,
> CREDIT UNION EXECUTIVES SOCIETY

"Your program was the highlight of our meeting. We have had nothing but favorable comments on your program, and I am more than happy to recommend it to other organizations as a sure fire winner of a program."
> John P. Seeley, President,
> AMERICAN SOCIETY OF ASSOCIATION EXECUTIVES

For information on having Dr. Teplitz speak to your group or organization, contact:
> Jerry Teplitz Enterprises, Inc.,
> 1304 Woodhurst Drive, Virginia Beach, VA 23454
> 800-777-3529 or 757-496-8008,
> Fax 757-496-9955
> Email Info@Teplitz.com
> www.Teplitz.com

YOUR MARKETPLACE: TOOLS FOR BETTER LIVING

SWITCHED-ON LIVING LEARNING SYSTEM

This book, (2) 45 minute DVDs and (4) CDs album is the same program that has been sold on TV by Dr. Jerry V. Teplitz. While other people talk about the power of positive thinking, Dr. Jerry V. Teplitz gives you the experience. He shows you how completely powerful YOU really are and how to apply that to all aspects of your life. He also focuses on the three key factors involved in living longer healthfully–Nutrition, Exercise, and Attitude. You will understand the things you can do to place yourself in charge of your own life. ($250)

TRAVEL STRESS: THE ART OF SURVIVING ON THE ROAD

This exciting six-CD audio album, with workbook, is designed to meet the needs of executives, managers, salespeople and anyone who spends time 'on the road'. Dr. Teplitz shares with you his proven travel techniques gathered from his years spent traveling as a professional speaker. ($95)

POWER OF THE MIND - DVD

Learn how completely powerful your mind is. Using your mind, you can actually create the things you want. Viewers will experience the difference between positive and negative thinking, how to change thought patterns, and the effects of music on the mind, body and performance. ($95)

INSTANT HEADACHE RELIEF - DVD

Just about everyone gets them. Now, there is a technique that is 2,000 years old which is both safe and effective called Shiatsu, a Japanese finger pressure technique for pain relief. Using it you can eliminate a headache (or a hangover) in 11/2 minutes and migraines in 5 minutes. This DVD also covers sinus colds, stiff necks, and sore shoulders. ($95)

YOUR SELLING SUCCESS FORMULA - CD

This four-CD audio album and self-assessment instrument allows you to become a more effective and successful salesperson by understanding your own selling behavior style as well as your clients' buying style. Companies have reported an increase in sales from 5-30%. ($85)

CREATING HIGH ENERGY WEB SITES AND PR MATERIALS - DVD

Your website and PR materials have an impact on your readers and surfers. The question is whether it is strengthening or weakening. If it's weakening, you get unintended consequences. This DVD of a live seminar will show you why and how you are impacting people and how to create a high energy product and website. ($150)

PAR AND BEYOND: SECRETS TO BETTER GOLF - DVD

This is a practical and dynamic DVD that shows you tools and techniques that immediately put you in charge of your game and will allow you to quickly and easily improve. You'll learn how to energize in seconds and refocus instantly. Golfers have reported playing their best game ever after watching this DVD. ($95)

SUBLIMINAL CD MUSIC

This series of CDs was designed by Steven Halpern to contain a unique process that uses music and inaudible positive statements to allow the listeners to achieve successful changes in their lives. Achieving Your Ideal Weight, Accelerating Learning, Enhancing Creativity, Enhancing Success, Enhancing Self-Esteem, Attracting Prosperity, Enhancing Creativity, Radiant Health and Well-Being, Success For Salespeople, Success For Managers. ($20)

To Order: Call 800 77-RELAX, 757-496-8008, Fax 757-496-9955, Email: Info@Teplitz.com, Website: www.Teplitz.com

JERRY V. TEPLITZ

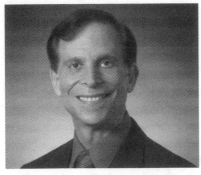

Jerry V. Teplitz is a graduate of Hunter College and Northwestern University School of Law. He also received his doctorate in Wholistic Health Sciences. He formerly practiced as an attorney with Illinois Environmental Protection Agency.

President of his own speaking and consulting firm since 1974, Dr. Teplitz conducts keynotes, seminars and training programs for associations, corporation and government agencies in the areas of stress management, management and leadership development, and sales success. He is also a certified consultant for The Inscape Publishing Company.

Besides authoring Managing Your Stress in Difficult Times, Dr. Teplitz has also written Switched-On Living and Brain Gym for Business. He has been the subject of articles in Prevention and numerous other magazines. He has appeared on over 300 radio and television shows throughout the United States and Canada, and has spoken to more than 1,000,000 people.

Dr. Teplitz earned the title of Certified Speaking Professional in 1982, which has been given by the National Speakers Association. This designation is held by less than 600 Speakers Worldwide. The Professional Convention Management Association selected him for their Best In Class Speaker Program. He's been listen in several editions of Who's Who in America.

SHELLY KELLMAN

Shelly Kellman was Senior Editor of Whole Life Times magazine. She is a freelance writer, photographer, graphic designer, publicist, and editorial consultant. Her articles have appeared in Whole Life Times, New Age, In These Times, Columbia University's Journal of International Affairs, and other publications. She has consulted or worked for the Illinois Department of Mental Health & Developmental Disabilities, the Cancer Prevention Center of Chicago, the Public Art Workshop (Chicago), the New York University School of Nursing, the Central America Education Fund (Boston), and numerous community and environmental organizations and private health professionals.